BODYWEIGHT WORKOUTS FOR SENIORS

BODYWEIGHT WORKOUTS FOR SENIORS

82 Zero-Equipment Functional Fitness Workouts to Strengthen Your Body, Coordinate Your Balance, and Energize Your Life

Sarah W. Jowers

CONTENTS

INTRODUCTION

Have you ever stumbled upon something unexpectedly, only to realize later that it would change your life forever? That's precisely how I came across the incredible world of bodyweight workouts for seniors. Allow me to share my personal story, one that ignited my passion for health and well-being and led me to discover the profound benefits of this fitness approach.

A few years ago, I found myself struggling with the common challenges that come with aging. My energy levels were plummeting, and I noticed a gradual decline in my strength, flexibility, and overall vitality. Feeling somewhat disheartened, I embarked on a journey to find a solution—a way to rejuvenate my body, mind, and spirit.

I had tried various workout programs in the past, but none seemed to fit my lifestyle or address the specific needs of seniors. Feeling determined, I dove deep into research, exploring different fitness modalities, until I stumbled upon a seemingly unassuming article about bodyweight workouts.

Curiosity sparked within me as I read about the incredible benefits that could be attained through these workouts. What intrigued me the most was the notion that I could harness the power of my body's natural strength and movements to achieve significant results. The idea of using my own body as a tool for transformation resonated deeply with me, and I knew I had found something special.

Eager to put my newfound knowledge into action, I began incorporating bodyweight workouts into my daily routine. To my amazement, I experienced noticeable improvements within weeks. My strength began to return, my flexibility increased, and I felt a renewed sense of vitality and confidence. These workouts were not only effective but also accessible, requiring no expensive equipment or gym memberships. I discovered that I could work out anytime, anywhere, at my own pace.

Excited by my personal progress and the immense potential I had uncovered, I dove deeper into the world of bodyweight workouts. I studied under expert trainers, explored countless variations and modifications, and delved into the science behind the movements. My passion grew, and it became clear that I had stumbled upon a goldmine of health and fitness for seniors.

As I shared my newfound knowledge and experiences with friends and family, I witnessed remarkable transformations in their lives as well. The sense of joy and fulfillment that came from helping others discover their own strength and regain their zest for life was unparalleled.

And now, here we are. This book, born out of my personal journey and the transformations I have witnessed, aims to guide you on your own path to strength, flexibility, mobility, coordination, balance, and cardiovascular endurance through the power of bodyweight workouts. Whether you're a senior seeking to regain vitality or a caregiver looking to support your loved ones, this book is designed to empower you.

In the following chapters, we will dive deep into the benefits of bodyweight workouts for seniors and provide you with a comprehensive guide to implementing these workouts into your daily life. We'll explore various workouts targeting different muscle groups, share expert tips on safety and progression, and provide sample workout plans to suit different fitness levels.

Let's embark on this journey together, as we embrace the transformative power of bodyweight workouts and cultivate a healthier, more vibrant life. Get ready to experience the joy of discovering what your body is truly capable of. Let's begin!

1. WHAT ARE BODYWEIGHT WORKOUTS?

Bodyweight workouts are workout routines that rely solely on the weight of your own body for resistance, without the need for additional equipment or weights. These workouts utilize a variety of movements and workouts that engage multiple muscle groups and promote strength, endurance, flexibility, and overall fitness.

With bodyweight workouts, you can perform workouts such as squats, push-ups, lunges, planks, and burpees, among many others. These workouts leverage the resistance provided by your body weight to challenge your muscles and improve your fitness levels. Bodyweight workouts are versatile, accessible, and can be modified to suit different fitness levels and abilities.

The beauty of bodyweight workouts lies in their convenience and accessibility. They can be done anywhere, anytime, making them a great option for individuals who prefer exercising at home, in a park, or while traveling. Moreover, bodyweight workouts require little to no equipment, making them cost-effective and suitable for those who don't have access to a gym or prefer a minimalist approach to fitness.

Why Bodyweight Workout?

In today's fast-paced world, it's easy for our health and well-being to take a backseat. As we age, the importance of maintaining a strong, flexible, and balanced body becomes increasingly evident. But what if I told you that achieving these goals doesn't require expensive gym memberships, bulky equipment, or complex workout routines. Here are some reasons why bodyweight workouts are well-suited for seniors:

Safety: Bodyweight workouts are generally low-impact and reduce the risk of injury compared to workouts that involve heavy weights or equipment. They allow you to engage in physical activity without putting excessive strain on your joints and muscles.

Convenience: The workouts can be done at home or in any suitable location without the need for specialized equipment or a gym membership. This convenience makes it easier for you to incorporate regular workout into your daily routine.

Functional Movement: Bodyweight workouts focus on movements that mimic everyday activities, such as squatting, bending, pushing, and pulling. By improving strength and mobility in these functional movements, you can enhance your ability to perform daily tasks and maintain independence.

Muscle Strength and Bone Health: Bodyweight workouts help you build and maintain muscle strength, which is crucial for maintaining balance, stability, and preventing age-related muscle loss (sarcopenia). Engaging in weight-bearing workouts also promotes bone health and reduces the risk of osteoporosis.

Joint Flexibility and Range of Motion: Bodyweight workouts involve movements that promote joint flexibility and improve range of motion. This can help you maintain or improve your joint health, reduce stiffness, and enhance overall mobility.

Cardiovascular Health: Many bodyweight workouts can be modified to increase heart rate and provide cardiovascular benefits. By incorporating movements that elevate the heart rate, such as jumping jacks or modified burpees, you can improve your cardiovascular endurance and maintain a healthy heart.

Customizability: Bodyweight workouts can be tailored to meet individual fitness levels and needs. You can start with basic workouts and gradually progress to more challenging variations as your strength and fitness improve.

How to Use this Book

This serves as a roadmap to help you make the most of the valuable content provided throughout the book. It is important to approach the book with an open mind and a willingness to embrace new ideas and concepts, as it is specifically designed for seniors, tailored to their unique needs and abilities.

Start by reading the introduction, which provides an overview of the book's content and sets the stage for what you can expect to gain from it. This will give you a sense of the overall structure and purpose of the book.

Each chapter focuses on a specific aspect of senior fitness, addressing topics such as preparing for success, assessing fitness levels, specific workouts for different body parts, flexibility and range of motion, cardiovascular health, and more. Take the time to understand the purpose and content of each chapter. Within each chapter, there are subchapters that delve deeper into specific topics. These subchapters provide detailed information on workouts, techniques, modifications, and progressions. Pay attention to these subchapters as they offer valuable insights and instructions.

The workout lists provided in each subchapter serve as a reference guide for different body parts and fitness goals. Take the time to familiarize yourself with these lists and choose workouts that align with your needs and abilities. Each workout comes with a detailed description that includes starting positions, movement explanations, muscle focus, breathing techniques, and recommended repetitions and sets. Study these descriptions carefully to ensure you understand how to perform each workout correctly and safely.

As you engage with the workouts, be open to modifications and progressions. Not everyone will start at the same fitness level, so it's important to listen to your body and adjust as needed. The book provides guidance on modifying workouts to suit your abilities and progressing as you build strength and stamina.

The book also offers guidance on designing a routine that fits your lifestyle and schedule. Consider your personal preferences, time constraints, and fitness goals when creating your workout plan. The sample workout plans provided can serve as a starting point for structuring your routine. It's always a good idea to consult with a healthcare professional or fitness expert, especially if you have any pre-existing medical conditions or concerns. They can provide personalized guidance and ensure that the workouts and routines align with your specific needs.

2. WARM-UP AND COOL-DOWN

In the realm of fitness, warm-up and cool-down routines are often overlooked, yet they play a vital role in optimizing your workout experience and preventing injuries.

A well-designed warm-up routine prepares your body for the upcoming physical activity by gradually increasing your heart rate, warming up your muscles, and improving your flexibility. It primes your body and mind for the workouts ahead, reducing the risk of strains, sprains, and other injuries.

On the other hand, cool-down routines are often neglected but are equally important. Cooling down allows your body to gradually return to its pre-workout state, gradually decreasing your heart rate and easing muscle tension. It helps prevent post-workout dizziness, soreness, and stiffness, while promoting relaxation and recovery. Incorporating a cool-down routine into your fitness routine can aid in reducing muscle fatigue and improve overall flexibility.

Before any bodyweight workouts in, it's crucial to warm up your body to prepare it for the physical activity ahead. A proper warm-up routine helps increase your heart rate, improves blood flow to your muscles, and enhances joint mobility. Here are some warm-up workouts and techniques for you:

Cardiovascular Warm-up: Start with five to ten minutes of light cardiovascular activity such as brisk walking, marching in place, or cycling on a stationary bike. This helps elevate your heart rate and increases blood circulation throughout your body.

Joint Mobilization: Perform gentle joint movements to lubricate your joints and increase their range of motion. Rotate your wrists, ankles, shoulders, and hips in a controlled and pain-free manner. Perform small circles or gentle swings to gradually warm up the joints.

Dynamic Stretching: Engage in dynamic stretching workouts that target the major muscle groups you'll be using during your bodyweight workout. Examples include arm circles, leg swings, and torso rotations. Perform each movement in a controlled manner, gradually increasing the range of motion as you warm up.

Bodyweight Movements: Incorporate light bodyweight movements that mimic the workouts you'll be performing in your workout. For example, perform bodyweight squats, lunges, or modified push-ups to activate the muscles and prepare them for the upcoming workouts.

Breathing Workouts: Practice deep breathing workouts to increase oxygen flow to your muscles and enhance relaxation. Take slow, deep breaths in through your nose, and exhale through your mouth. Focus on filling your lungs completely and exhaling fully.

Cool-down

After completing your bodyweight workout routine, it's essential to engage in a proper cool-down to gradually bring your body back to a resting state. Cooling down allows your heart rate and breathing to return to normal, helps prevent muscle soreness, and promotes recovery. Here are some effective cool-down techniques for you:

Gentle Cardiovascular Activity: Transition from your workout to a lower-intensity cardiovascular activity, such as slow walking or light cycling. Perform this activity for about five to ten minutes to gradually decrease your heart rate and cool down your body.

Static Stretching: Engage in static stretching workouts to improve flexibility and release tension in the muscles. Focus on stretching the major muscle groups that were targeted during your workout. Hold each stretch for 15 to 30 seconds, without bouncing or straining, and remember to breathe deeply.

Deep Breathing and Relaxation: Take a few moments to practice deep breathing and relaxation techniques. Inhale deeply through your nose, and exhale slowly through your mouth. Focus on releasing any remaining tension in your body and promoting a sense of relaxation and calmness.

Self-Massage or Foam Rolling: Use a foam roller or your hands to perform gentle self-massage on the areas that feel tense or tight. Apply light pressure and roll or massage the muscles to alleviate any discomfort and promote muscle recovery.

Hydration: Drink water to rehydrate your body after the workout. It's important to replenish fluids lost during workout to support proper bodily functions and aid in recovery.

3. UPPER BODY STRENGTH AND MOBILITY

Our arms, chest, back, and shoulders play vital roles in supporting daily activities and maintaining overall functionality. This chapter will guide you through a series of workouts specifically designed to target these areas, helping you build strength, improve mobility, and enhance your overall quality of life.

In today's modern world, many of us spend hours sitting at desks or engaging in activities that primarily involve our lower body. As a result, our upper body muscles can become weak and stiff, limiting our range of motion and hindering our ability to perform tasks with ease. However, with the right workouts and consistent effort, we can unlock the potential of our upper body, promoting strength, flexibility, and increased functionality.

Arm Workouts

These workouts target the muscles in your arms, helping you improve strength, tone, and flexibility. Remember to warm up before starting these workouts

Arm Circles

Starting position: Stand with your feet shoulder-width apart. Extend your arms straight out to the sides at shoulder height, parallel to the ground. Keep your palms facing down.

Movement description:

Begin by making small circular motions with your arms. Imagine drawing circles in the air with your fingertips. Gradually increase the size of the circles, making sure to maintain control and proper form throughout the movement. You can choose to rotate your arms clockwise or counterclockwise.

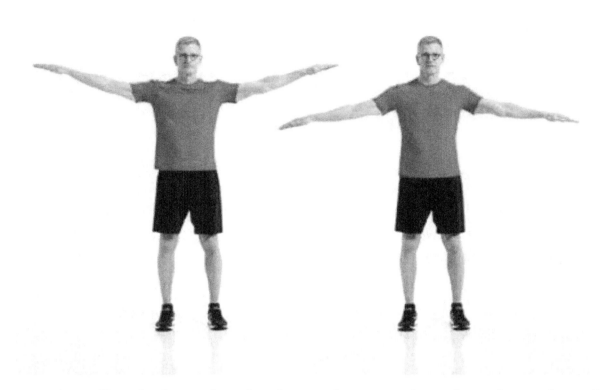

Breathing: Breathe in a relaxed and natural manner throughout the workout. Inhale and exhale slowly and steadily without holding your breath.

Repetitions and sets: Start with a comfortable number of repetitions, such as 10-15 arm circles in each direction. As you become more comfortable and confident, gradually increase the number of repetitions or the duration of the workout. Aim for 2-3 sets of arm circles.

* If you find it challenging to perform the workout with your arms fully extended, you can slightly bend your elbows to reduce the range of motion.

Chair Dips

Starting position: Sit on the edge of a sturdy chair with your hands placed on the chair's seat on either side of your hips. Keep your feet flat on the floor, hip-width apart, and knees bent at a 90-degree angle.

Movement description: Slide your hips forward off the chair, supporting your weight with your hands. Keep your fingers pointing forward and grip the chair firmly. With your back close to the chair, slowly lower your body towards the floor by bending your elbows. Lower yourself until your elbows are at a 90-degree angle or slightly lower.

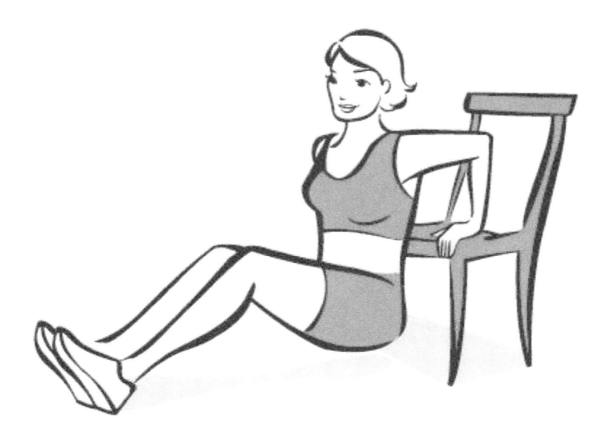

Breathing: Inhale as you lower your body towards the floor, and exhale as you push back up to the starting position.

Repetitions and sets: Start with a comfortable number of repetitions, such as 8 to 10. Aim for 2 to 3 sets of chair dips. Gradually increase the number of repetitions and sets as you get stronger and more comfortable with the workout.

Modifications:

To make chair dips easier: Place your feet closer to the chair, which will decrease the amount of body weight you need to lift. You can also keep your knees bent throughout the workout to reduce the load on your arms.

To make chair dips more challenging: Extend your legs in front of you, keeping your heels on the floor. This increases the weight you need to lift and adds more resistance to the workout. You can also elevate your feet on a higher surface, such as another chair or step, to intensify the workout.

Wall Push-Ups

Starting Position: Stand facing a wall at arm's length. Place your hands on the wall at shoulder height, slightly wider than shoulder-width apart. Step back a comfortable distance, keeping your feet hip-width apart. Ensure your body is in a straight line from head to heels.

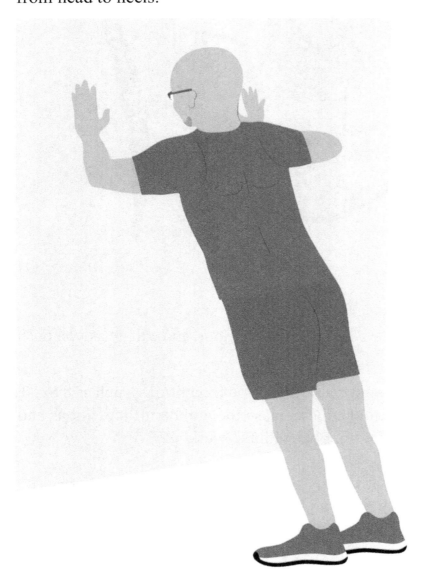

Movement Description:

Inhale and engage your core muscles.

Lower your chest towards the wall by bending your elbows, while keeping your body straight and your heels on the ground.

Exhale and push away from the wall by straightening your arms, returning to the starting position.

Breathing: Inhale before you begin the movement, exhale as you push away from the wall.

Repetitions and Sets: Start with a comfortable number of repetitions, such as 8 to 10, and gradually increase as you become stronger. Aim for 2 to 3 sets of wall push-ups.

Modifications and Progressions:

To make the workout easier: Stand closer to the wall, reducing the angle of your body. This decreases the resistance and makes the workout less challenging.

To make the workout more challenging: Step further away from the wall, increasing the angle of your body. This increases the resistance and intensifies the workout.

Overhead Arm Raises

Starting position: Stand with your feet shoulder-width apart and your arms down by your sides.

Movement description: Slowly raise both arms straight out in front of you, keeping them parallel to the ground. Continue raising your arms overhead until they are fully extended, reaching towards the ceiling. Maintain a controlled and smooth movement throughout.

Breathing: Inhale as you lower your arms down by your sides, and exhale as you raise your arms overhead.

Repetitions and sets: Start with a comfortable number of repetitions, such as 8 to 10 repetitions. Perform 2 to 3 sets of the workout. As you become more comfortable and stronger, you can gradually increase the number of repetitions and sets.

Modified version: If raising both arms overhead simultaneously is challenging, you can try raising one arm at a time. Lift one arm up towards the ceiling while keeping the other arm down by your side, then alternate arms for each repetition.

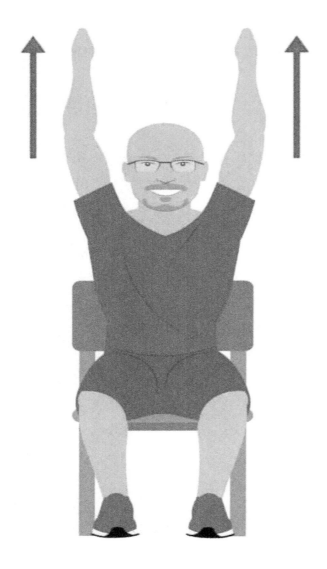

Wrist Rotations

Starting Position: Sit comfortably in a chair with your feet flat on the floor and your back straight.

Extend your arms forward, parallel to the ground, with your palms facing down.

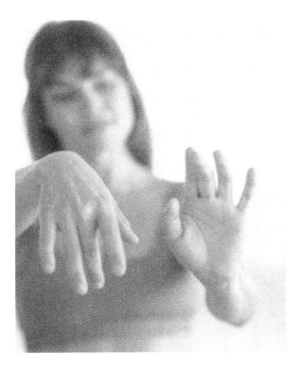
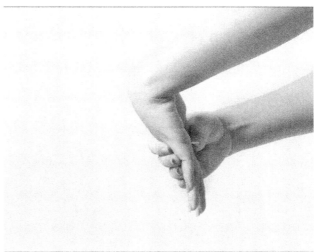

Movement Description:

Begin by slowly rotating your wrists in a circular motion.

Start with small circles, and gradually increase the size of the circles as you feel more comfortable.

Perform the rotations in a controlled manner, avoiding any sudden or jerky movements.

Continue the rotation for the desired number of repetitions.

Breathing:

Breathe in a relaxed and natural manner throughout the workout. Inhale and exhale steadily, without holding your breath.

Repetitions and Sets:

Start with 10 repetitions in each direction (clockwise and counterclockwise). As you progress, you can gradually increase the number of repetitions or perform multiple sets with a short rest in between.

Modifications: If you find it challenging to perform the wrist rotations with both arms simultaneously, you can start by focusing on one arm at a time.

Finger Extension

Starting Position:

Sit comfortably in a chair or on a stable surface.

Rest your forearm on a table or your thigh, with your palm facing down.

Keep your fingers relaxed and extended straight.

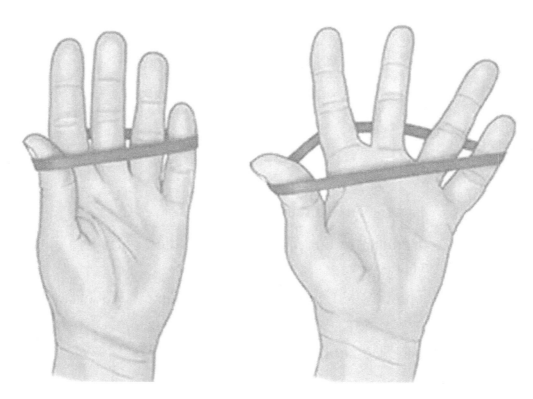

Movement Description:

Slowly lift each finger, one at a time, off the table or your thigh.

Extend each finger as far as possible, spreading them apart.

Maintain control and avoid excessive tension or strain.

Repetitions and Sets:

Aim to perform 10 to 15 repetitions of the finger extension workout.

Start with a comfortable number of repetitions and gradually increase over time.

Complete 2 to 3 sets of the workout, resting briefly between sets.

Modifications:

If you find it challenging to lift each finger individually, you can start by lifting two or three fingers together and gradually work towards lifting each finger independently.

Plank Shoulder Taps

Starting Position: Begin by getting into a plank position. Place your hands directly under your shoulders on the floor/mat, keeping your arms straight.

Extend your legs straight behind you, resting on your toes. Keep your body in a straight line from your head to your heels, engaging your core muscles.

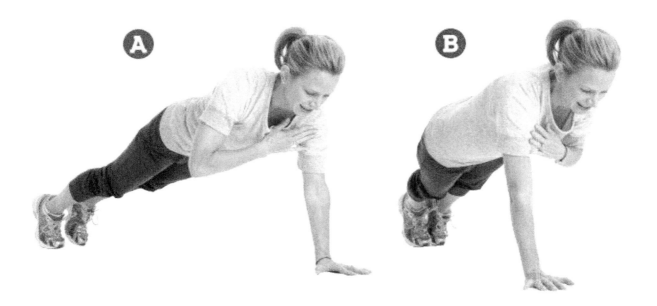

Movement Description:

While maintaining the plank position, lift one hand off the floor and tap the opposite shoulder gently.

Place the hand back down on the floor, and repeat the same action with the other hand, tapping the opposite shoulder.

Continue alternating shoulder taps, maintaining a stable plank position throughout the workout.

Breathing:

Inhale deeply before starting the movement.

Exhale as you tap the shoulder, engaging your core muscles and maintaining stability.

Inhale again as you return the hand to the starting position.

Repetitions and Sets:

Start with a comfortable number of repetitions, such as 5-8 taps on each shoulder.

Gradually increase the number of repetitions as you build strength and endurance.

Aim to perform 2-3 sets of the workout, resting briefly between sets.

Modifications and Progressions:

If the full plank position is challenging, you can modify by performing the workout with your knees resting on the floor instead of being on your toes. This is known as a modified plank.

As you gain strength and stability, progress to performing the workout in a full plank position, supporting your body weight on your toes.

To make the workout more challenging, you can increase the tempo of the shoulder taps or add a slight lift of the foot on the opposite side as you tap the shoulder.

Wall Diamond Push-Ups

Starting Position: Stand facing a wall and position your hands at chest level against the wall, forming a diamond shape with your thumbs and index fingers. Step back a comfortable distance from the wall, ensuring your feet are hip-width apart and your body is in a straight line.

Movement Description:

Bend your elbows and lower your chest toward the wall while keeping your body straight. Focus on maintaining control and a slow, controlled pace throughout the movement. Lower yourself until your chest is close to the wall, then push yourself back up to the starting position by extending your arms.

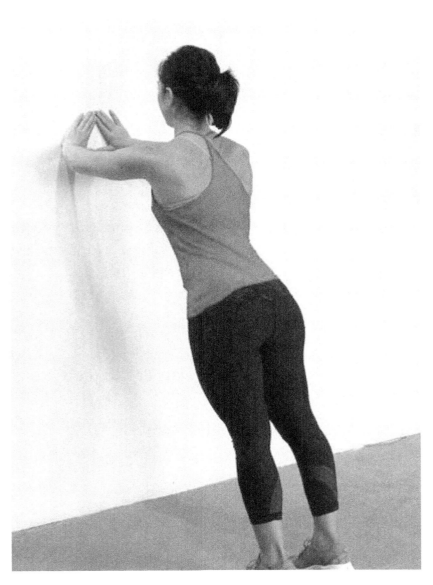

Breathing:

Inhale as you lower your chest toward the wall and exhale as you push yourself back up to the starting position. Remember to breathe steadily throughout the workout.

Repetitions and Sets:

Start with a manageable number of repetitions, such as 8 to 10 repetitions. As you become more comfortable and stronger, gradually increase the number of repetitions or sets. Aim for 2 to 3 sets of wall diamond push-ups.

Modifications and Progressions:

You can modify this workout by standing closer to the wall, which reduces the amount of body weight being lifted. This modification makes the workout easier while still engaging the targeted muscles. To progress, you can gradually step back from the wall, increasing the angle and difficulty of the workout.

Chest Workouts

Let's explore a variety of bodyweight workouts specifically designed for you to target the chest muscles without the need for any equipment. These workouts are safe, effective, and can be performed in the comfort of your own home.

Chest Opener

Starting Position:

Stand with your feet shoulder-width apart and your arms extended to the sides at shoulder height.

Ensure that your palms are facing forward and your shoulders are relaxed.

Movement Description:

Slowly bring your arms forward, crossing them in front of your chest.

Imagine you are giving yourself a gentle hug as you cross your arms.

Open your arms back out to the sides, returning to the starting position.

Maintain a controlled and smooth motion throughout the workout.

Breathing:

Inhale as you open your arms out to the sides, expanding your chest. Exhale as you bring your arms forward and cross them in front of your chest.

Repetitions and Sets:

Start with a manageable number of repetitions, such as 8 to 10 repetitions. Gradually increase the number of repetitions as you become more comfortable and stronger. Aim for 2 to 3 sets of Chest Openers during your workout session.

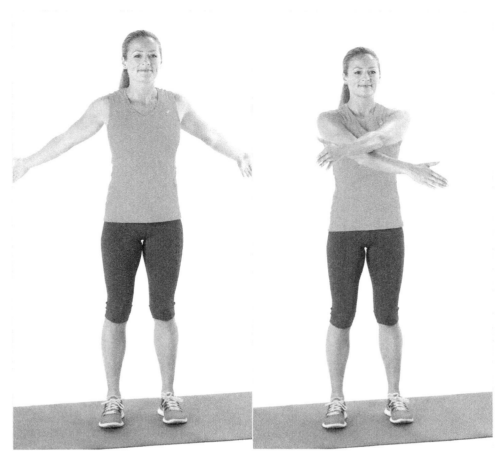

Modification: If you find it challenging to cross your arms in front of your chest, simply bring your arms forward without crossing them. Focus on opening your arms out to the sides and returning to the starting position.

Arm Hugs

Starting Position:

Stand with your feet shoulder-width apart and maintain an upright posture.

Extend your arms out to the sides at shoulder height, keeping your palms facing forward.

Movement Description:

Slowly bring your arms forward, crossing them in front of your chest.

As you cross your arms, imagine giving yourself a gentle hug, feeling the stretch across your chest.

Open your arms back out to the sides, returning to the starting position.

Repeat the movement in a controlled manner.

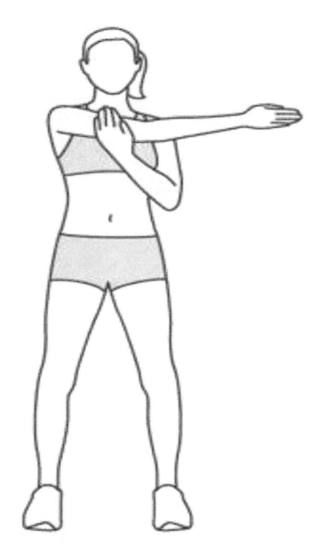

Breathing:

Inhale as you open your arms out to the sides, and exhale as you bring your arms forward to cross them in front of your chest.

Repetitions and Sets:

Start with a manageable number of repetitions, such as 8 to 10 repetitions. Gradually increase the number of repetitions as you become more comfortable and stronger. Aim for 2 to 3 sets of Arm Hugs during your workout session.

Modifications: If you find it challenging to bring your arms all the way across your chest, you can start with a smaller range of motion, gradually increasing it as your chest muscles become more flexible.

Incline Push-Ups

Starting Position:

Find a stable elevated surface like a sturdy bench, countertop, or step.

Place your hands slightly wider than shoulder-width apart on the elevated surface.

Position your body at an angle, leaning forward with your feet together and your toes on the ground.

Keep your body straight, engage your core, and maintain a neutral spine position.

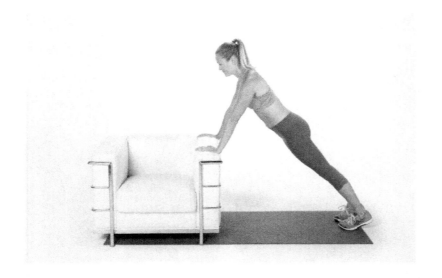

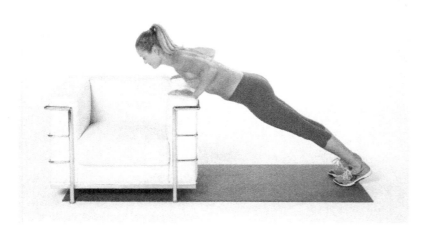

Movement Description:

Lower your chest towards the elevated surface by bending your elbows.

Maintain control and keep your body aligned as you descend.

Lower yourself until your chest is just above the elevated surface or as far as you can comfortably go.

Push yourself back up by straightening your arms, returning to the starting position.

Focus on controlling the movement and engaging your chest muscles throughout the workout.

Breathing:

Inhale as you lower your chest towards the elevated surface, and exhale as you push yourself back up to the starting position. Maintain a steady breathing rhythm throughout the workout.

Repetitions and Sets:

Start with a comfortable number of repetitions that you can perform with proper form. Aim for 8-12 repetitions in each set. Gradually increase the number of sets as you progress and build strength.

Modifications:

If the incline push-ups are too challenging initially, you can increase the angle by using a higher elevated surface, such as a wall, and gradually work your way down to a lower surface.

To make the workout easier, you can perform incline push-ups against a countertop or wall, adjusting the angle to suit your current fitness level.

Bear Hugs

Starting Position: Stand tall with your feet shoulder-width apart and your arms relaxed by your sides or sit on a chair

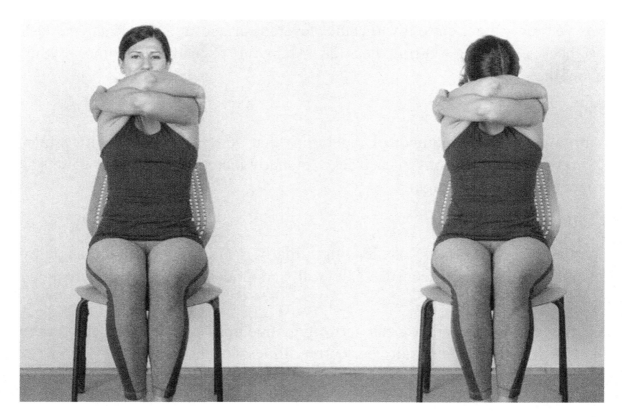

Movement Description: Extend your arms straight out in front of you at shoulder height. Keeping your arms extended, open them wide, as if you're giving someone a big bear hug. Then, bring your arms back together in front of your chest.

Repetitions and Sets: Start with 10 repetitions and aim to complete 2 to 3 sets. Rest for 30 seconds to 1 minute between sets.

Modifications:

For a lighter intensity, perform smaller arm movements by not extending your arms as far out or bringing them as close together.

Standing/Seated Chest Press

Starting Position:

Stand with your feet shoulder-width apart and knees slightly bent or sit on chair.

Extend your arms straight out in front of you, palms facing forward and at shoulder height.

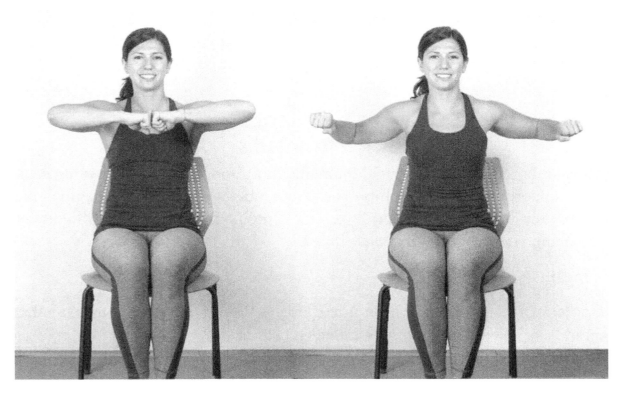

Movement Description:

Push your hands forward, bringing them closer together as if you're pressing against an imaginary resistance.

Keep your elbows slightly bent throughout the movement to engage your chest muscles.

Control the movement and avoid any sudden or jerky motions.

Repetitions and Sets:

Start with a comfortable number of repetitions, such as 8-12 repetitions.

Gradually increase the number of repetitions as you become more comfortable and stronger.

Aim for 2-3 sets of this workout, with a brief rest period between sets.

Modifications:

If you find the workout challenging, you can decrease the intensity by bringing your hands slightly closer together or performing the movement with a slower tempo.

As you progress, you can also increase the number of sets or incorporate variations of the workout, such as standing on one leg to challenge your balance.

Back Workouts

A strong and flexible back is essential for maintaining good posture, preventing back pain, and supporting overall mobility. These workouts will help you strengthen the muscles in your upper, middle, and lower back, promoting better spinal alignment and enhancing your overall functional fitness.

Superman

Starting Position: Lie face down on a mat or the floor, with your arms extended straight in front of you and your legs extended behind you.

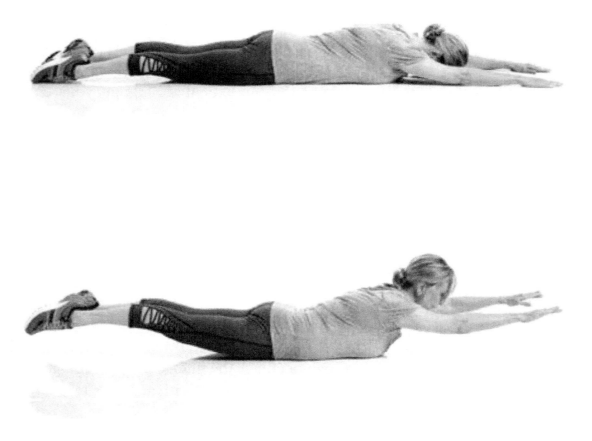

Movement: Simultaneously lift your arms, chest, and legs off the floor, engaging your back muscles. Imagine reaching your arms and legs away from your body as if you were flying like Superman.

Muscle Focus: Targets the muscles of the upper and lower back, including the erector spinae, rhomboids, and trapezius.

Breathing: Inhale as you prepare for the movement, and exhale as you lift your arms, chest, and legs off the floor.

Repetitions and Sets: Start with 8 to 10 repetitions and 2 to 3 sets. Gradually increase the number of repetitions and sets as your strength improves.

Modifications:

To make it easier: Keep your legs on the ground and only lift your upper body, focusing on squeezing your back muscles.

To make it more challenging: Lift your arms, chest, and legs higher off the floor and hold the position for a few seconds before lowering down.

Bird Dog

Starting Position: Begin on your hands and knees, with your hands aligned under your shoulders and knees under your hips.

Movement: Extend your right arm forward while simultaneously extending your left leg backward. Keep your spine neutral and avoid arching your back. Hold the position for a moment, then return to the starting position and repeat on the opposite side.

Breathing: Inhale as you prepare, exhale as you extend your arm and leg, and inhale as you return to the starting position.

Repetitions and Sets: Perform 8 to 10 repetitions on each side for 2 to 3 sets.

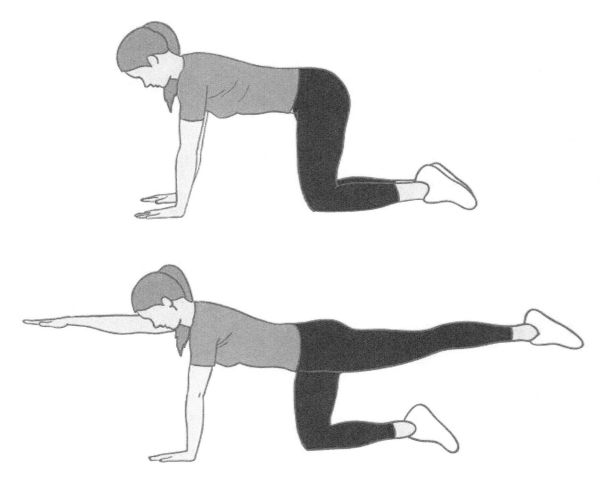

Modifications:

Beginner: If balancing on hands and knees is challenging, you can start by lifting one arm or leg at a time instead of doing the full bird dog movement. Focus on maintaining stability and control.

Intermediate: As you become more comfortable with the workout, you can increase the duration of the hold at the extended position. Aim to hold for a few seconds longer on each repetition.

Advanced: To add more challenge, you can lift the opposite arm and leg simultaneously, creating a longer lever. This requires greater balance and stability.

Bridge

Starting Position: Lie on your back with your knees bent and feet flat on the ground, hip-width apart. Place your arms by your sides, palms facing down.

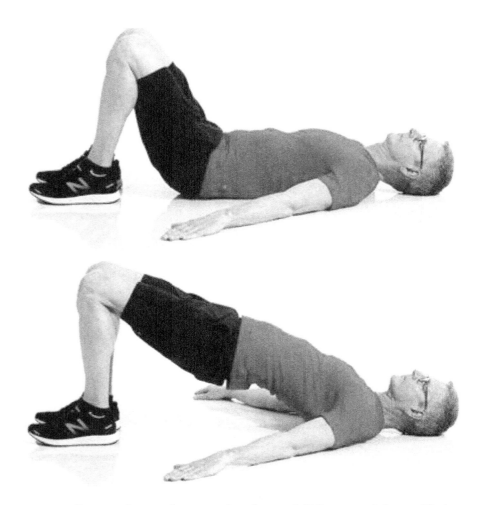

Movement: Press through your heels and lift your hips off the ground, creating a straight line from your knees to your shoulders. Squeeze your glutes and engage your core.

Breathing: Inhale as you prepare, exhale as you lift your hips, and inhale as you lower them back down.

Repetitions and Sets: Aim for 10 to 12 repetitions and 2 to 3 sets.

Modifications:

Beginner: If lifting your hips off the ground is challenging, start by lifting only a few inches and gradually increase the range of motion as you get stronger.

Advanced: To make the workout more challenging, try single-leg bridges. Lift one foot off the ground while maintaining the bridge position, then switch legs after a set of repetitions.

Progressive: As you become more comfortable with the workout, you can add a pause at the top of the bridge, holding the position for a few seconds before lowering down.

Prone Back Extension

Starting Position: Lie face down on the floor with your legs extended and your arms resting alongside your body

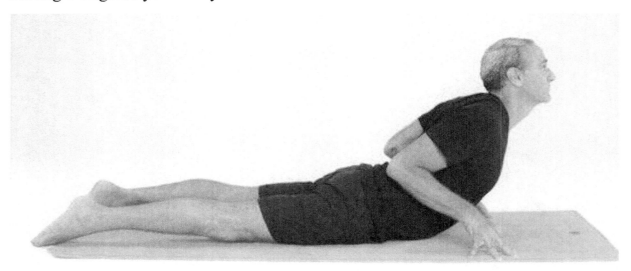

Movement Description: Keeping your neck aligned with your spine, slowly lift your chest off the floor while maintaining a gentle contraction in your glutes (buttocks). Lift until you feel a comfortable stretch in your lower back but avoid hyperextension.

Muscle Focus: Targets the muscles of the lower back, including the erector spinae.

Breathing: Inhale as you prepare for the movement, and exhale as you lift your chest off the floor.

Repetitions and Sets: Aim for 8 to 12 repetitions and perform 2 to 3 sets.

Modifications: If you find the workout challenging, you can start by lifting your chest only slightly off the floor and gradually increase the range of motion as you build strength. For a more advanced variation, you can place your hands behind your head or lightly clasp them behind your back

Cobra Stretch

Starting Position: Lie face down on the floor with your legs extended and toes pointed. Place your hands on the floor under your shoulders, fingers pointing forward.

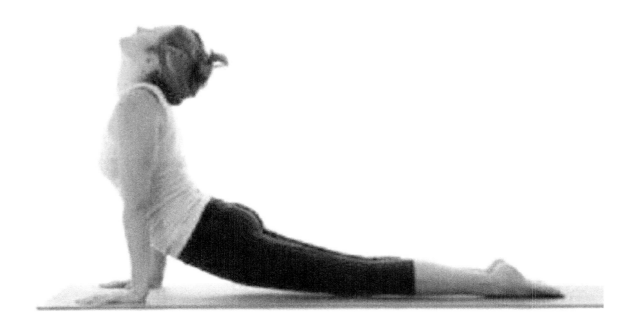

Movement: Press your palms onto the floor and slowly lift your upper body, keeping your hips and legs grounded. Arch your back and lift your chest as high as comfortably.

Breathing: Inhale as you prepare, and exhale as you lift your chest.

Repetitions and Sets: Hold the stretch for 15 to 30 seconds and repeat for 2 to 3 sets.

Modifications and Progressions:

If you have limited flexibility, you can perform a modified cobra stretch by propping yourself up on your forearms instead of fully extending your arms.

For a deeper stretch, you can lift your thighs off the floor slightly while keeping your hips grounded.

As you progress, you can gradually increase the duration of the stretch and the number of repetitions.

Standing Back Extension

Starting position: Stand upright with your feet shoulder-width apart and your hands resting on the back of your hips or crossed over your chest.

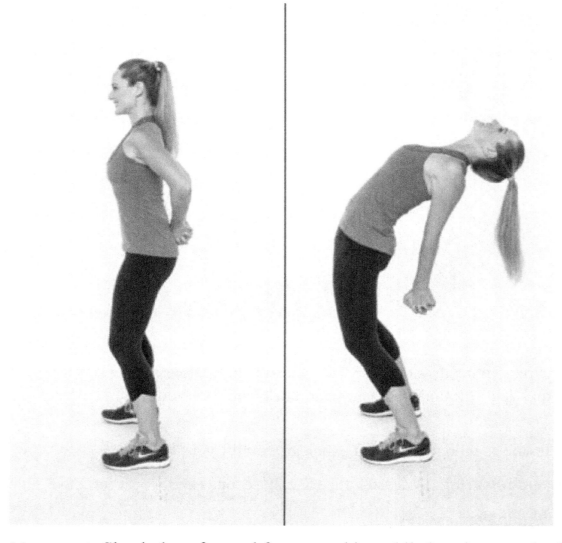

Movement: Slowly lean forward from your hips while keeping your back straight, allowing your upper body to tilt forward. Engage your core muscles and squeeze your shoulder blades together as you lean back, extending your spine. Return to the starting position by reversing the movement, gently tilting forward again.

Breathing: Inhale as you prepare to lean forward, exhale as you lean back, and inhale as you return to the starting position.

Repetitions and Sets: Start with 8 to 10 repetitions and aim for 2 to 3 sets. Gradually increase the repetitions or sets as you become more comfortable and stronger.

Modifications:

For beginners or those with limited mobility, perform the workout with a smaller range of motion, focusing on maintaining proper form and engaging the back muscles.

To increase the challenge, you can place your hands on the back of your head, keeping your elbows wide. This will add additional resistance and engage the muscles of the upper back and shoulders.

Wall Slide

Starting Position:

Stand with your back against a wall, with your feet shoulder-width apart and about a foot away from the wall. Your back, hips, and head should all be in contact with the wall. Relax your arms by your sides.

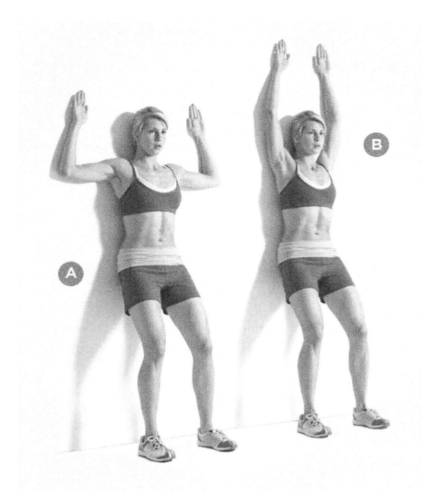

Movement Description:

Slowly slide your arms up the wall while keeping them in contact with the wall. Continue sliding your arms until they are overhead, maintaining contact with the wall throughout the movement.

As you slide your arms up, focus on squeezing your shoulder blades together. Imagine that you are trying to pinch a pencil between them.

Pause briefly at the top position, feeling the stretch in your chest and upper back.

Slowly lower your arms back down the wall to the starting position, maintaining contact with the wall throughout the movement.

Breathing:

Inhale as you prepare to slide your arms up the wall. Exhale as you slide your arms up, focusing on squeezing your shoulder blades together. Inhale as you pause at the top position, and exhale as you lower your arms back down.

Repetitions and Sets:

Start with 8 to 10 repetitions of the wall slide workout. Gradually increase the number of repetitions as you feel more comfortable and gain strength. Aim for 2 to 3 sets.

Modifications:

If you find the workout challenging, you can start by standing closer to the wall and sliding your arms up a shorter distance.

To increase the intensity, you can hold a slight contraction at the top position for a couple of seconds before lowering your arms back down.

Reverse Snow Angels

Starting position:

Lie on your stomach with your arms extended above your head and your palms facing down on the floor.

Your legs should be straight and together, with your toes pointed down.

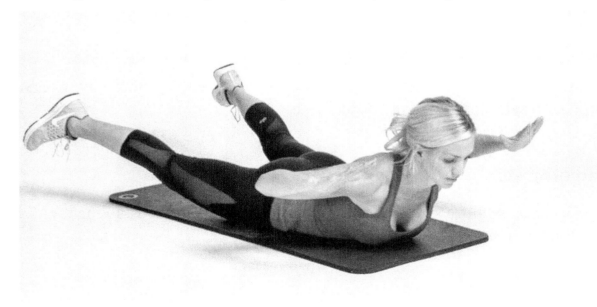

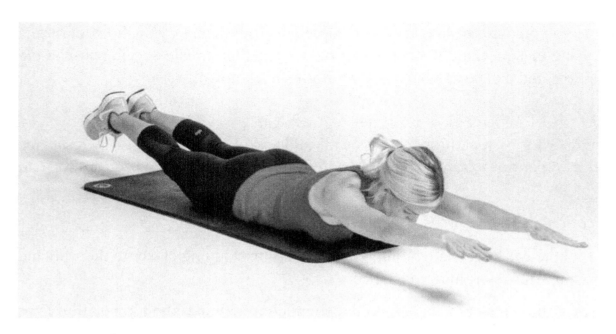

Movement description:

Keeping your arms straight, lift them up and out to your sides, forming a "Y" shape with your body.

Hold for a second or two, then lower your arms back down to the starting position.

Breathing: Inhale as you lift your arms up and exhale as you lower them back down.

Repetitions and sets:

Start with 2 sets of 10 repetitions, and gradually increase the number of repetitions as you get stronger.

Modifications:

If you find this workout too difficult, you can start by bending your elbows and keeping your hands closer to your body.

Cat-Camel Stretch

Starting Position: Begin on your hands and knees, with your hands aligned under your shoulders and knees under your hips.

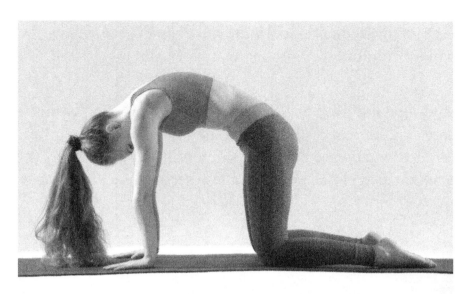

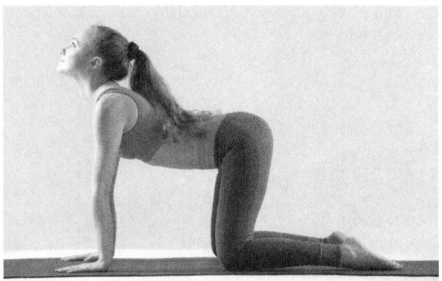

Movement: Arch your back upward like a cat, then lower it downward and lift your chest like a camel. In the cat position, round your back upward, tuck your chin towards your chest, and allow your head to drop slightly. Feel the stretch in your upper back and between your shoulder blades. In the camel position, lower your belly towards the floor, lift your chest, and extend your head and neck, looking upward. Feel the stretch in your lower back and front of your body.

Breathing: Inhale as you prepare to move, exhale as you round your back into the cat position, and inhale as you arch your back into the camel position. Focus on deep, slow breaths to enhance relaxation and movement.

Repetitions and Sets: Repeat the movement 8 to 10 times, gradually increasing the repetitions as you become more comfortable with the workout. Aim to perform 2 to 3 sets.

Modifications: If you have limited mobility or flexibility, move gently and within a comfortable range that allows you to feel a stretch without any pain or discomfort. As you progress, you can gradually increase the range of motion and the duration of each position, holding the cat and camel positions for a few seconds longer.

Plank

Starting Position: Begin by lying face down on the floor. Position your elbows directly under your shoulders and place your forearms on the ground. Extend your legs back so you are balanced on your toes.

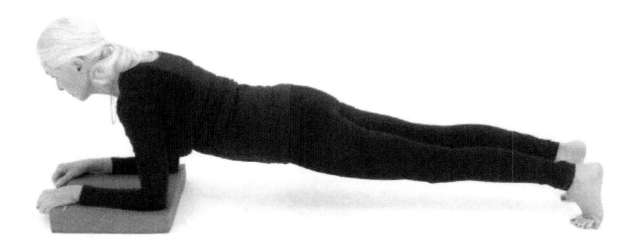

Movement Description: Lift your body off the ground, keeping your back and legs straight. Engage your core muscles and avoid sagging or arching your back. Your body should form a straight line from your head to your heels.

Breathing: Breathe evenly and deeply throughout the workout. Inhale and exhale naturally, without holding your breath.

Repetitions and Sets: Start with holding the plank position for 20 to 30 seconds, focusing on maintaining proper form and engaging the targeted muscles. As you progress, gradually increase the duration to 45 seconds, 1 minute, or longer, according to your comfort level.

Modifications: If the full plank is challenging, you can modify the workout by performing a forearm plank, where you balance on your forearms instead of your hands. To make the workout easier, you can also perform the plank with your knees on the ground. As you become stronger, you can progress to more challenging variations, such as side planks or plank variations with leg lifts or arm movements.

Shoulder Workouts

The shoulders play a crucial role in many daily activities, such as reaching, lifting, and carrying objects. As we age, it becomes even more important to maintain strong and mobile shoulders to support our independence and overall well-being.

Through a series of bodyweight workouts, we will target the muscles surrounding the shoulder joint, including the deltoids, rotator cuff muscles, and upper back muscles. These workouts will help enhance your shoulder stability, range of motion, and overall functional ability.

Shoulder Rolls

Starting Position: Stand tall with your feet shoulder-width apart, maintaining good posture. Relax your arms by your sides.

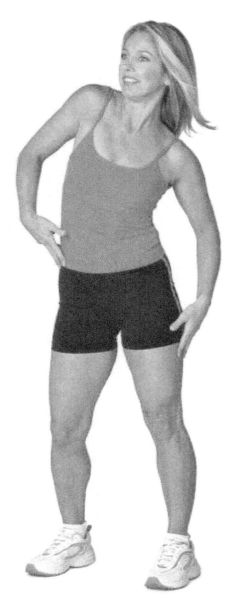

Movement Description: Begin by rolling your shoulders forward in a circular motion. Lift your shoulders up towards your ears, then roll them forward and down in a smooth and controlled manner. Continue the circular motion, allowing your shoulder blades to move freely.

Breathing: Inhale as you lift your shoulders up, and exhale as you roll them forward and down.

Repetitions and Sets: Start with 8 to 10 shoulder rolls in one direction, then reverse the direction and perform another 8 to 10 rolls. Aim to complete 1 to 2 sets of this workout.

Modifications: If you have limited mobility or shoulder discomfort, you can perform smaller shoulder rolls or reduce the range of motion. If you feel comfortable with the movement, you can increase the number of repetitions or sets gradually.

Prone Y Raises

Starting Position:

Lie face down on the floor or a workout mat, with your arms extended overhead and your legs straight.

Keep your forehead resting on the mat and engage your core muscles.

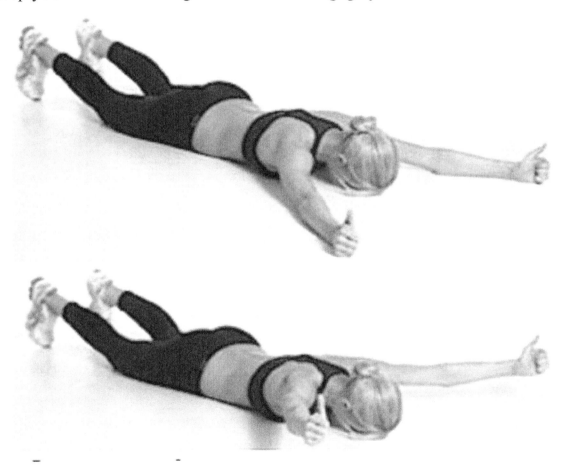

Movement Description:

Inhale and engage your shoulder blades by squeezing them together.

Exhale as you lift your chest, arms, and head off the ground simultaneously, forming a Y shape with your body.

Focus on keeping your neck in a neutral position, looking towards the floor.

Keep your arms straight and palms facing down throughout the movement.

Breathing:

Inhale as you prepare for the movement. Exhale slowly and steadily as you lift your chest, arms, and head off the ground. Inhale as you lower back down to the starting position.

Repetitions and Sets:

Start with a comfortable number of repetitions, such as 8 to 10 repetitions. Gradually increase the number of repetitions as you become more comfortable and stronger. Aim for 2 to 3 sets of Prone Y Raises.

Modifications:

If you find it challenging to lift your chest, arms, and head off the ground simultaneously, you can start by lifting one arm at a time while keeping the other arm resting on the ground.

As you progress, you can also increase the range of motion by lifting your arms higher and focusing on squeezing your shoulder blades together.

Prone T Raises

Starting Position:

Lie face down on the floor, extending your body fully. Keep your legs straight and together and place your forehead on the ground.

Extend your arms out to the sides, forming a T shape with your body. Palms should be facing down, and your thumbs should point towards the ceiling.

Movement Description:

Engage your core and squeeze your glutes to stabilize your body.

Lift your chest, arms, and head off the ground simultaneously. Keep your gaze down to maintain proper neck alignment.

As you lift, focus on squeezing your shoulder blades together and feeling the muscles in your upper back engage.

Maintain a slight bend in your elbows throughout the movement.

Pause briefly at the top of the movement, feeling the contraction in your shoulder blades.

Slowly lower your chest, arms, and head back down to the starting position.

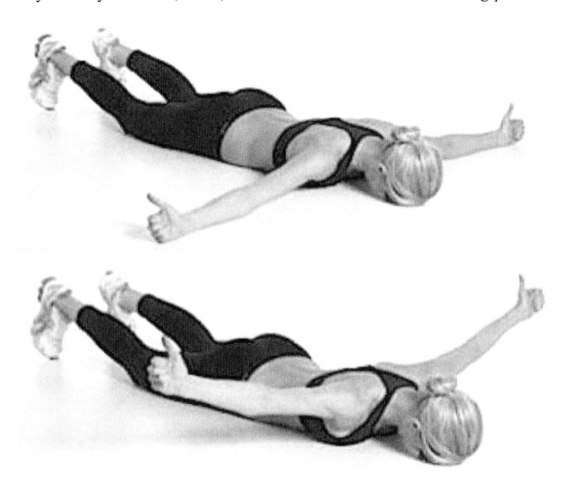

Breathing:

Inhale as you lower your chest, arms, and head towards the ground. Exhale as you lift your chest, arms, and head off the ground.

Repetitions and Sets:

Start with 8-10 repetitions of Prone T Raises. Gradually increase the number of repetitions as you become more comfortable and stronger. Aim to perform 2-3 sets of this workout.

Modifications:

If you find it challenging to lift your chest and arms off the ground, you can perform a modified version by lifting only your chest and keeping your arms on the ground.

Arm Reaches

Starting Position:

Stand tall with your feet hip-width apart.

Relax your shoulders and keep your spine in a neutral position.

Extend your arms down by your sides, with palms facing your thighs.

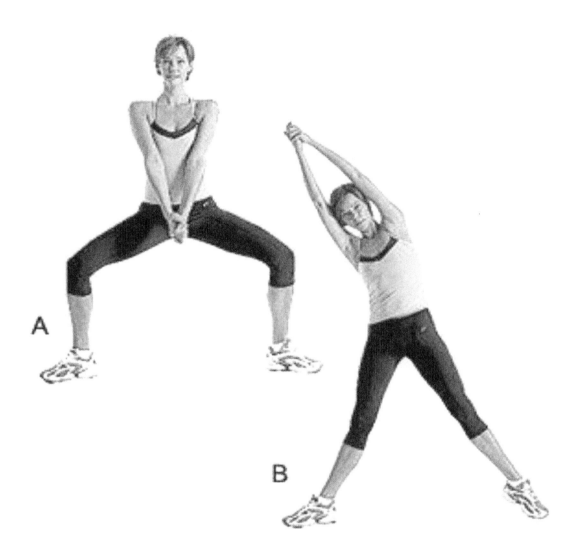

A

B

Movement Description:

Begin by lifting one arm straight overhead, reaching towards the opposite side.

Keep your arm straight but avoid locking your elbow.

Maintain a controlled and smooth movement throughout.

Feel the stretch and lengthening in your side body and shoulder as you reach.

Breathing:

Inhale as you prepare to reach.

Exhale as you perform the reaching motion.

Repetitions and Sets:

Start with 8-10 repetitions on each side.

Gradually increase the number of repetitions as you feel comfortable.

Aim for 2-3 sets of the workout.

Modifications:

If reaching overhead is challenging, you can modify the workout by performing a lower reach to the side, gradually increasing the range of motion as you gain strength and flexibility.

To progress the workout, you can add a gentle side bend towards the reaching arm, engaging your core muscles for stability and further enhancing the stretch.

Shoulder Circles

Starting Position: Stand tall with your feet shoulder-width apart. Relax your arms by your sides.

Movement Description: Begin by lifting your shoulders up towards your ears in a circular motion. Slowly roll your shoulders back, squeezing your shoulder blades together. Continue the circular motion by bringing your shoulders down and forward, completing the circle. Repeat the movement in the opposite direction.

Breathing: Inhale as you lift your shoulders up towards your ears and exhale as you roll them back and down.

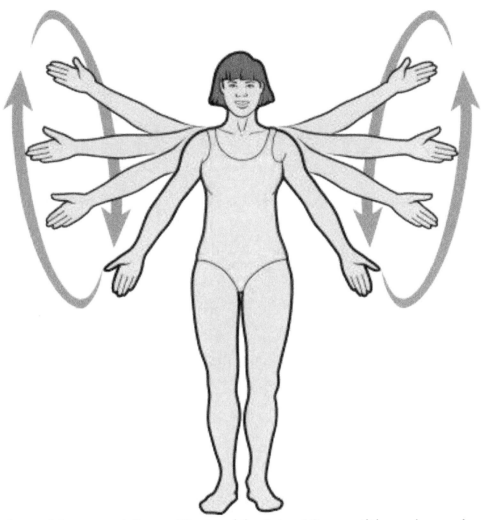

Repetitions and Sets: Start with 5 to 10 repetitions in each direction, gradually increasing as you become more comfortable and stronger. Aim for 2 to 3 sets.

Modifications:

Modified Shoulder Circles: If standing is uncomfortable or challenging, you can perform shoulder circles while sitting on a chair or stability ball. Maintain an upright posture and follow the same circular motion with your shoulders.

Range of Motion: Adjust the size of the circles based on your comfort level. Start with smaller circles and gradually increase the range of motion as your shoulders become more flexible and mobile.

Arm Position: You can modify the workout by extending your arms out to the sides while performing shoulder circles. This will provide additional resistance and engage the muscles of the arms.

Tempo Variation: To add variety, you can perform shoulder circles at different tempos. Slow down the movement to focus on control and stability or increase the speed to challenge your coordination and endurance.

Pike Push-Ups

Starting Position:

Begin in a push-up position with your hands slightly wider than shoulder-width apart and your feet together.

Walk your feet forward, raising your hips into an inverted "V" shape. Keep your arms and legs straight.

Adjust the position of your hands to ensure your wrists are directly under your shoulders.

Movement Description:

Bend your elbows and lower your upper body toward the floor, bringing your head towards the ground.

As you lower yourself down, maintain a controlled movement and engage your shoulder muscles.

Once your head is close to the ground or at a comfortable level, push through your hands to raise your body back up to the starting position.

Focus on keeping your core engaged and maintaining a straight line from your head to your hips throughout the movement.

Breathing:

Inhale as you lower your upper body towards the ground.

Exhale as you push through your hands to raise your body back up to the starting position.

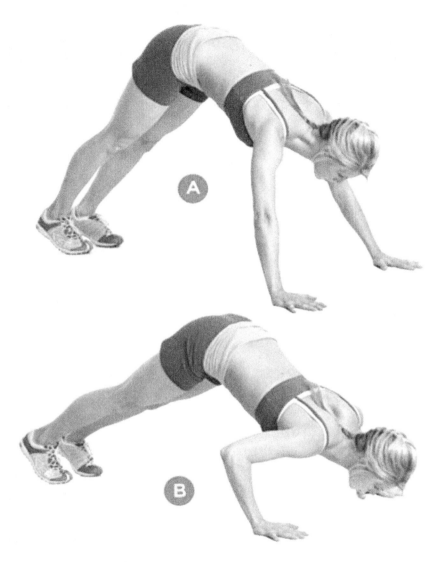

Repetitions and Sets:

Start with a number of repetitions that are challenging but manageable for you, such as 8-10 reps.

Aim to complete 2-3 sets of Pike Push-Ups, resting for 1-2 minutes between sets.

As you become more comfortable and stronger, you can gradually increase the number of repetitions or sets.

Modifications:

To make Pike Push-Ups easier: Instead of having your feet together, spread them slightly wider for a more stable base of support. You can also perform the workout with your hands elevated on a stable surface, such as a bench or step, to decrease the intensity.

To make Pike Push-Ups more challenging: Increase the range of motion by lowering your head closer to the ground. You can also try performing the workout with your feet elevated on a sturdy object, such as a step or chair, to increase the difficulty.

Overhead Arm Claps

Starting Position:

Stand with your feet shoulder-width apart, maintaining good posture with your back straight and shoulders relaxed.

Extend your arms straight out to the sides, parallel to the floor, with your palms facing down.

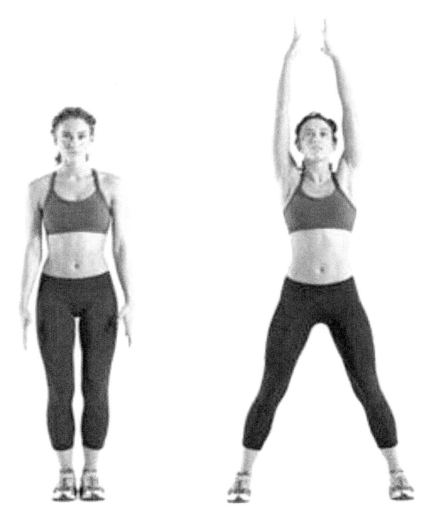

Movement Description:

Begin by bringing your arms together in front of your body, extending them overhead.

As your arms reach the overhead position, gently clap your hands together.

Open your arms wide, bringing them back to the starting position with palms facing down.

Breathing:

Inhale as you bring your arms together and lift them overhead.

Exhale as you open your arms wide and return to the starting position.

Repetitions and Sets:

Start with a comfortable number of repetitions, such as 8 to 10.

Gradually increase the number of repetitions as you become more comfortable and stronger.

Aim to perform 2 to 3 sets of this workout, resting for a short period between sets.

Modifications:

If you find it challenging to perform this workout with straight arms, you can slightly bend your elbows.

Doorway Stretch

Starting Position:

Stand in a doorway, facing forward.

Raise your right arm to a 90-degree angle, placing your forearm and palm against the doorframe at shoulder height.

Step forward slightly with your right foot, allowing your chest to be in line with the doorframe.

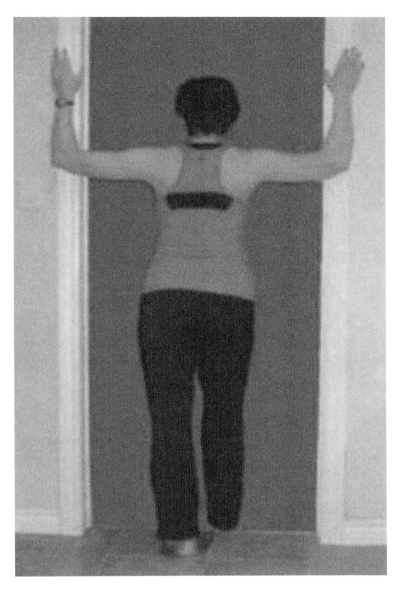

Movement Description:

Gently lean forward, shifting your weight onto your front foot, while keeping your arm and hand pressed against the doorframe.

As you lean forward, you should feel a gentle stretch across the front of your right shoulder and chest.

Hold the stretch for 20-30 seconds, maintaining a comfortable position without any sharp pain or discomfort.

Relax and release the stretch, slowly stepping back to the starting position.

Repeat the stretch on the opposite side, raising your left arm and leaning forward to stretch the left shoulder and chest.

Breathing:

Throughout the workout, remember to breathe deeply and naturally. Inhale slowly and deeply before starting the stretch, and exhale gently as you lean forward into the stretch. Maintain relaxed breathing throughout the hold.

Repetitions and Sets:

Perform the Doorway Stretch for each side (right and left) once, holding the stretch for 20-30 seconds on each side. You can repeat the stretch for multiple sets if desired, ensuring you take short rest periods between sets.

Modifications:

If you find it challenging to step forward and lean into the stretch, you can perform the stretch without stepping, simply standing in a comfortable position and pressing your arm against the doorframe to feel the stretch.

To progress the stretch, you can slightly increase the lean forward, while maintaining control and without compromising your balance or comfort. Gradually increase the intensity of the stretch over time as your flexibility improves.

4. LOWER BODY STRENGTH AND FLEXIBILITY

In this chapter, we will dive into the realm of lower body strength and flexibility, unlocking the potential for improved mobility, balance, and overall well-being. The lower body plays a crucial role in our daily activities, from walking and climbing stairs to maintaining stability and independence.

As we age, it becomes increasingly important to prioritize the strength and flexibility of our lower body muscles. The workouts in this chapter are carefully selected to cater to different fitness levels and address common concerns such as leg strength, hip mobility, and ankle stability.

Leg Workouts

Our legs are the foundation of our mobility, allowing us to walk, climb, and perform daily activities with ease. By engaging in specific workouts that target legs, we can improve overall leg function, boost endurance, and support our active lifestyles.

Squats

Starting position: Stand with your feet hip-width apart, toes slightly turned out for comfort. Engage your core by pulling your belly button toward your spine. Keep your chest lifted and maintain a neutral spine throughout the workout.

Movement description:

Bend your knees and lower your body as if sitting back into an imaginary chair. Keep your weight on your heels and your knees aligned with your toes. Descend until your thighs are parallel to the ground, or as low as you can comfortably go. Avoid letting your knees extend past your toes.

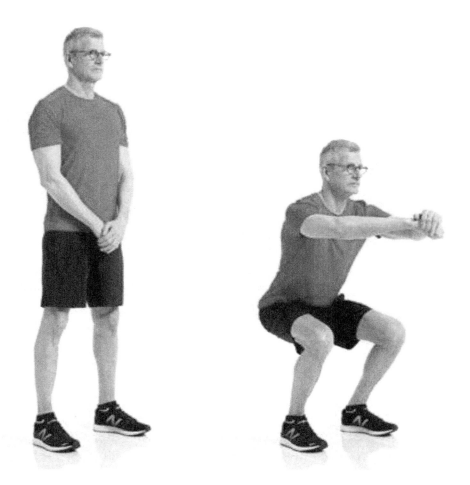

Breathing: Inhale as you lower your body and exhale as you push through your heels to stand back up.

Repetitions and sets: Start with a manageable number of repetitions, such as 8-10, and gradually increase as you build strength and confidence. Aim for 2-3 sets of squats.

Modifications:

If you find it challenging to perform a full squat, you can use a chair for support. Stand in front of the chair with your feet hip-width apart, slowly lower your body until you touch the chair with your buttocks, and then stand back up. As you gain strength, you can gradually reduce the height of the chair until you can perform a full squat.

Lunges

Starting position: Stand with your feet hip-width apart and your hands on your hips or relaxed by your sides.

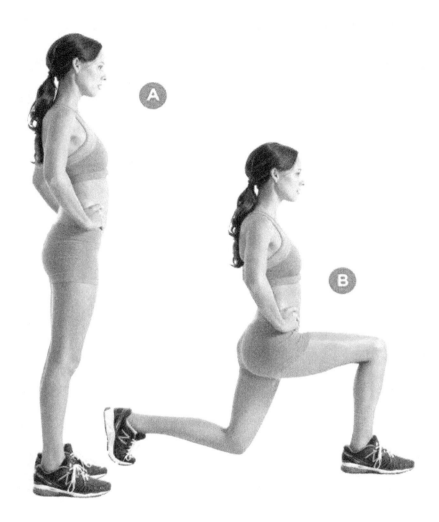

Movement description:

Step forward with your right foot, taking a comfortable stride length. Keep your upper body upright and engage your core for stability.

Lower your body by bending both knees until your front knee is directly above your ankle and your back knee is hovering just above the ground. Aim to create a 90-degree angle with both knees.

Pause for a moment in the lowered position, maintaining proper alignment and balance.

Push through your front heel and engage your leg muscles to return to the starting position.

Repeat the movement with your left leg stepping forward, alternating between right and left legs.

Breathing: Inhale as you step forward and prepare to lower your body. Exhale as you push through your front heel to return to the starting position.

Repetitions and sets: Start with a comfortable number of repetitions, such as 8-10 lunges per leg. Gradually increase the number of repetitions as you feel stronger. Aim for 2-3 sets of lunges, resting for a short period between sets.

Modifications:

Chair-assisted lunges: Hold onto a chair or wall for support while performing the lunges to enhance stability.

Reverse lunges: Instead of stepping forward, step backward with one leg while keeping the same movement and muscle focus.

Walking lunges: Perform lunges by taking forward steps, walking across a room or along a designated path.

Step-ups

Starting position: Stand facing a step or elevated surface, ensuring it is sturdy and secure. Place your feet hip-width apart.

Movement description: Step one foot onto the elevated surface, ensuring your entire foot is on the step. Push through the heel of the raised foot and engage your leg muscles to bring your other foot up onto the step. Both feet should now be on the step. Step back down, leading with the same foot you started with. Repeat the movement, alternating the leading foot with each repetition.

Breathing: Inhale as you step up, exhale as you step down.

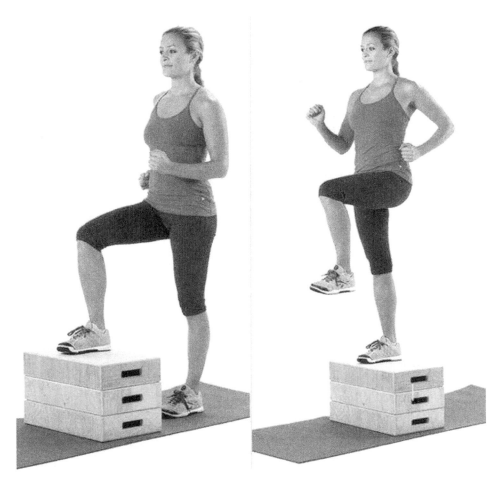

Repetitions and sets: Start with a comfortable number of repetitions, such as 8 to 10 on each leg, and aim to complete 2 to 3 sets. Gradually increase the number of repetitions and sets as your strength and endurance improve.

Modification: If stepping onto a high step feels challenging, start with a lower step or platform and gradually work your way up to a higher step as you gain strength and confidence.

Calf Raises

Starting Position:

Stand with your feet hip-width apart near a wall or chair for support.

Engage your core muscles and maintain an upright posture throughout the workout.

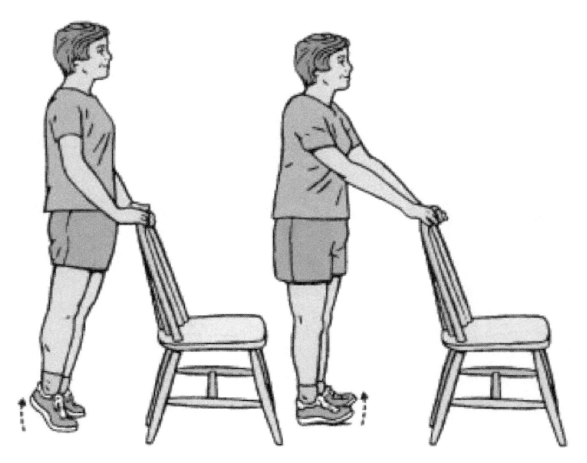

Movement Description:

Slowly lift your heels off the ground, rising onto the balls of your feet.

Focus on pushing through the balls of your feet and lifting your heels as high as possible.

Hold the raised position for a moment, feeling the contraction in your calf muscles.

Slowly lower your heels back down to the starting position.

Muscle Focus:

Calf raises primarily target the calf muscles, specifically the gastrocnemius and soleus muscles. These muscles are responsible for ankle flexion and provide strength and stability for walking, running, and maintaining balance.

Breathing:

Inhale as you lower your heels to the starting position, and exhale as you lift your heels off the ground.

Repetitions and Sets:

Start with a comfortable number of repetitions, such as 10 to 12 repetitions for each set. Aim to gradually increase the number of repetitions as your strength improves. Perform 2 to 3 sets of calf raises.

Modifications:

If you find it challenging to balance on both feet, you can perform calf raises while holding onto a sturdy surface, such as a wall or chair.

To increase the difficulty, perform the workout on one leg at a time, lifting the opposite foot off the ground.

To add variety, you can perform calf raises on an elevated surface, such as a step or curb, allowing your heels to drop below the level of the platform for a deeper stretch.

Wall Sits

Starting position:

Stand with your back against a wall.

Position your feet slightly wider than hip-width apart, about a foot or so away from the wall.

Ensure your back is in contact with the wall throughout the workout.

Movement description:

Slowly slide your back down the wall, bending your knees.

Continue sliding down until your knees are bent at a 90-degree angle, or as close to 90 degrees as feels comfortable for you.

Ideally, your thighs should be parallel to the ground.

Maintain a neutral spine and engage your core throughout the workout.

Hold this position for the desired duration.

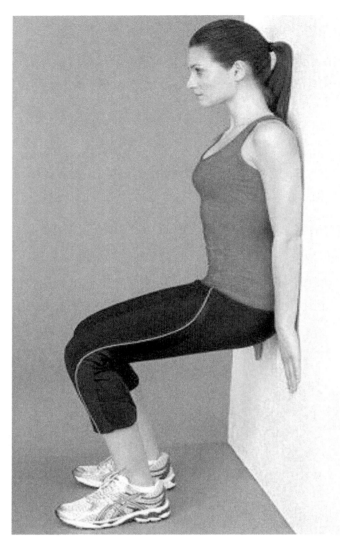

Breathing:

Inhale deeply before lowering yourself into the wall sit position.

Exhale gradually as you lower yourself down and hold the position.

Breathe steadily and maintain a consistent breathing pattern throughout the exercise

Repetitions and sets:

Start with holding the wall sit position for around 10-20 seconds.

Gradually increases the duration as your strength and endurance improve.

Aim to perform 2-3 sets of wall sits during your workout session.

Modifications:

If the 90-degree knee bend is too challenging, you can start with a slightly higher position and gradually progress to a deeper wall sit.

If you feel discomfort or strain in your knees or lower back, try adjusting your position by bending your knees to a more comfortable angle.

For an added challenge, you can lift one foot off the ground and hold the wall sit position with one leg.

Standing Leg Swings

Starting position:

Stand near a wall or chair for support. Place your feet shoulder-width apart and maintain a good posture with your head up and shoulders relaxed.

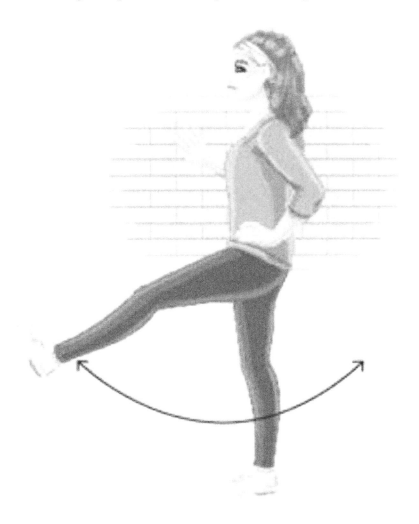

Movement description:

Shift your weight onto one leg and slightly bend that knee.

Engage your core muscles to maintain stability and balance throughout the workout.

Keeping your leg straight or slightly bent at the knee, swing your other leg forward and backward in a controlled manner.

Allow your leg to swing freely, finding a comfortable range of motion. Avoid excessive force or jerky movements.

Control the swinging motion with your leg muscles, rather than relying on momentum.

Breathing:

Breathe naturally throughout the workout. Inhale and exhale in a relaxed manner, focusing on maintaining a steady breathing rhythm.

Repetitions and sets:

Start with a comfortable number of repetitions, such as 8 to 10 swings per leg. Gradually increase the repetitions as you become more comfortable and confident. Aim for 2 to 3 sets of leg swings on each leg.

Modifications:

If balance is a concern, hold onto a wall or chair with one hand for additional support while performing the swings.

Progression: As you gain strength and stability, try increasing the range of motion of the leg swings by gradually swinging your leg higher.

Side Leg Raises

Starting position:

Stand near a wall or chair for support.

Stand with your feet hip-width apart and engage your core for stability.

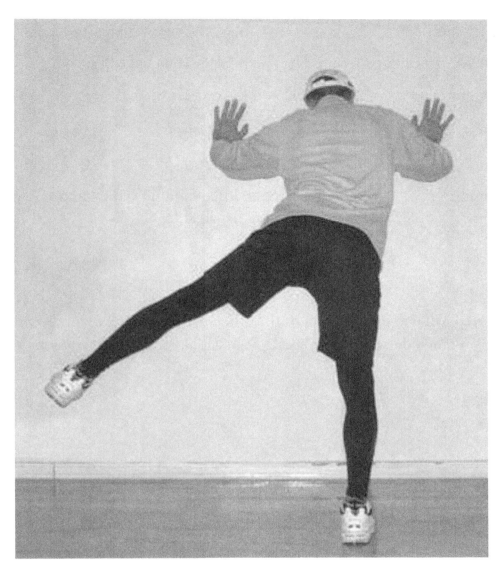

Movement description:

Lift one leg out to the side, keeping it straight or slightly bent at the knee.

Keep your toes pointing forward and maintain a slight bend in the opposite leg for balance.

Avoid leaning or tilting your upper body; instead, stay upright and focus on the movement of your leg.

Breathing:

Breathe in as you lift your leg to the side.

Exhale as you lower your leg back down to the starting position.

Repetitions and sets:

Begin with a comfortable number of repetitions, such as 8-10 on each side.

Gradually increase the number of repetitions as you become stronger.

Aim for 2-3 sets of side leg raises during your workout session.

Modifications:

If you find it challenging to perform side leg raises while standing, you can modify the workout by sitting on a chair and lifting your leg to the side.

Heel-To-Toe Walk

Starting position: Stand with one foot in front of the other, touching heel to toe. Keep your arms relaxed by your sides or lightly rest on a wall or chair for support if needed.

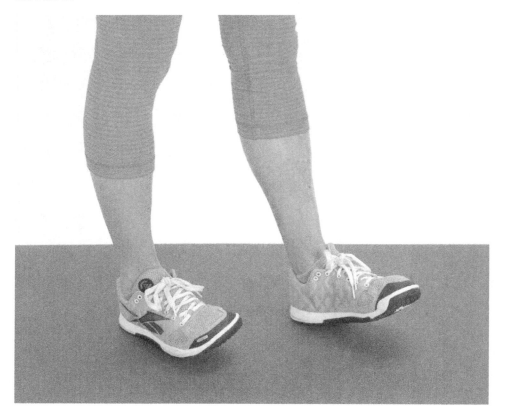

Movement description: Take small steps, maintaining heel-to-toe contact. Focus on transferring your weight smoothly from your heel to the toe of the opposite foot with each step. Keep your gaze forward and maintain good posture throughout the workout.

Breathing: Breathe naturally throughout the workout, maintaining a relaxed and steady breathing pattern. Inhale and exhale in a comfortable manner that feels natural to you.

Repetitions and sets: Start with a distance that feels comfortable for you, such as walking in a straight line for about 10-15 steps. Gradually increase the distance as you feel more confident and stable. Aim to perform 2-3 sets of the heel-to-toe walk during each workout session.

Modifications: If you find it challenging to maintain balance while walking heel-to-toe, you can use a wall, chair, or a sturdy object for support. As you gain more stability, gradually reduce the reliance on support until you can perform the workout without assistance. To progress the workout, you can try performing the heel-to-toe walk on different surfaces, such as grass or sand, which will further challenge your balance and coordination.

Ankle Circles

Starting position: Sit on a chair with your feet lifted off the ground.

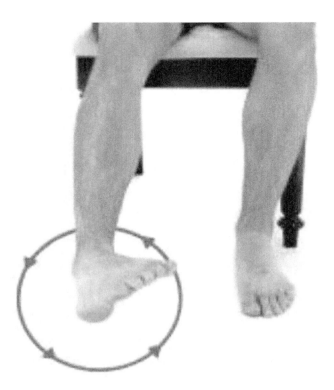

Movement description: Begin by extending one leg in front of you, keeping it relaxed. Slowly rotate your ankle in a circular motion. Perform a set number of circles in one direction, then switch and rotate the ankle in the opposite direction. Make sure to perform the movement in a controlled and smooth manner.

Breathing: Breathe in a relaxed and controlled manner throughout the workout. Maintain a steady breathing rhythm.

Repetitions and sets: Start with 5 to 10 circles in each direction for each ankle. Gradually increase the number of repetitions as you feel more comfortable and capable. Aim for 2 to 3 sets of ankle circles during your workout session.

Modifications: If you have difficulty sitting on a chair, you can perform ankle circles while lying down on your back. You can also perform ankle circles with one leg crossed over the other, adding a slight stretch to the calf muscles.

Hip Workouts

The hips play a crucial role in our everyday activities, from walking and sitting to maintaining balance and stability. As we age, it becomes even more important to prioritize hip strength and flexibility to support our overall mobility and quality of life.

Hip Marching

Starting position: Stand tall with your feet hip-width apart. Place your hands on your hips or use a chair or wall for support if needed.

Movement description: Lift one knee up towards your chest while keeping your back straight. Engage your core muscles to maintain stability and balance throughout the movement. Hold the lifted position for a brief moment.

Breathing: Inhale as you prepare to lift your knee and exhale as you lift it towards your chest. Maintain a steady breathing pattern throughout the workout.

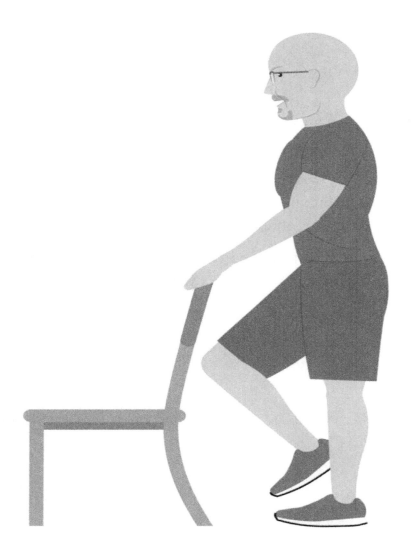

Repetitions and sets: Start with a comfortable number of repetitions, such as 8 to 10 on each leg. Gradually increase the repetitions as you feel stronger and more comfortable. Aim for 2 to 3 sets of the workout.

Modifications: If you have difficulty lifting your knee high, you can start with smaller movements and gradually work your way up to higher knee lifts. Using a chair or wall for support can also help with balance and stability.

Standing Hip Extensions

Starting Position:

Stand behind a chair or any stable support, maintaining an upright posture.

Place your feet hip-width apart, with your toes pointing forward.

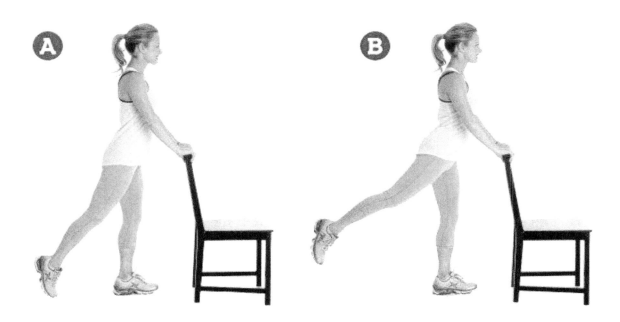

Movement Description:

Shift your weight onto one leg, while keeping the knee slightly bent.

Engage your core muscles for stability and balance.

Slowly lift the other leg straight back behind you, maintaining a straight line from your head to your heel.

Keep your feet flexed and toes pointing downward throughout the movement.

Pause briefly at the top of the movement, feeling the contraction in your glute muscles.

Slowly lower your leg back down to the starting position.

Breathing:

Inhale as you prepare for the movement. Exhale as you lift your leg and engage your glutes. Inhale again as you lower your leg back down.

Repetitions and Sets:

Start with 8 to 10 repetitions on each leg, and gradually increase the number of repetitions as your strength improves. Aim for 2 to 3 sets.

Modifications:

If you find it challenging to maintain balance, hold onto a chair or wall for support until you feel more confident.

To increase the difficulty, try extending your leg further back or holding the end position for a longer duration.

Clamshells

Starting Position:

Lie on your side on a comfortable surface, such as a mat or carpet.

Bend your knees slightly, keeping your feet together.

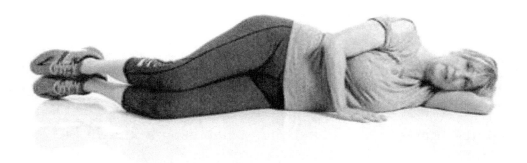

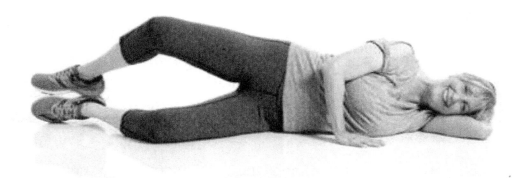

Movement Description:

While maintaining the bend in your knees, slowly lift your top knee as high as you comfortably can, while keeping your feet together.

Focus on using your hip muscles to lift the leg, rather than relying on momentum.

Muscle Focus:

The Clamshells workout primarily targets the muscles in your hips, specifically the gluteus medius and gluteus minimus.

Repetitions and Sets:

Start with a comfortable number of repetitions, such as 8 to 10 repetitions on each side. Gradually increase the number of repetitions as you become more comfortable with the workout. Aim for 2 to 3 sets.

Modifications:

If you find it challenging to keep your feet together, you can place a small foam or cushion between your knees to provide additional support.

Standing Hip Abduction

Starting position: Stand tall with your feet hip-width apart. Place your hands on your hips or hold onto a sturdy chair or wall for support.

Movement description: Lift one leg out to the side, keeping it straight and toes pointing forward. Try to maintain good balance and control throughout the movement.

Muscle focus: The primary muscles targeted in this workout are the hip abductors, including the gluteus medius and gluteus minimus. These muscles are responsible for moving your leg away from the midline of your body.

Breathing: Inhale as you prepare for the movement, and exhale as you lift your leg out to the side.

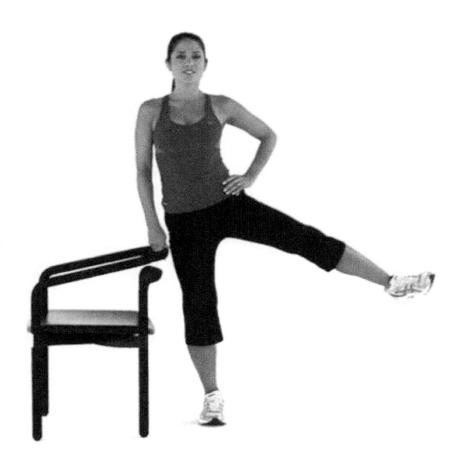

Repetitions and sets: Start with a comfortable number of repetitions, such as 8-10 repetitions per leg. Gradually increase the number of repetitions as you become more comfortable and stronger. Aim for 2-3 sets of this workout.

Modifications: If you find it challenging to perform the workout while standing, you can modify it by holding onto a chair or wall for support.

Seated Leg Extensions

Starting position: Sit on a chair with your back straight and feet flat on the ground. Place your hands on the sides of the chair for support.

Movement description: Extend one leg forward, keeping it straight and parallel to the ground. Engage your thigh muscles as you extend your leg. Hold this position briefly, feeling the tension in your thigh muscles.

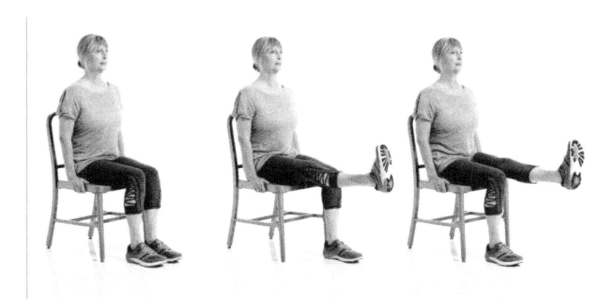

Breathing: Inhale as you prepare to extend your leg. Exhale as you extend your leg and engage your muscles. Inhale as you return to the starting position.

Repetitions and sets: Start with a comfortable number of repetitions, such as 8 to 10 repetitions per leg. Aim to gradually increase the number of repetitions as your strength improves. Perform 2 to 3 sets of leg extensions, resting briefly between sets.

Modifications: If you find it challenging to fully extend your leg, you can start by bending your knee slightly and gradually work towards straightening it. Additionally, you can increase the difficulty of this workout by adding ankle weights or holding a water bottle or small weighted object between your feet.

Fire Hydrants

Starting position: Begin on your hands and knees on a comfortable mat or soft surface. Place your hands directly below your shoulders and your knees directly below your hips. Keep your spine in a neutral position, with a slight natural curve.

Movement description: Engage your core muscles to stabilize your body. Lift one knee out to the side, keeping your knee bent at a 90-degree angle. Imagine mimicking the movement of a dog lifting its leg to hydrant. Your thigh should be parallel to the ground.

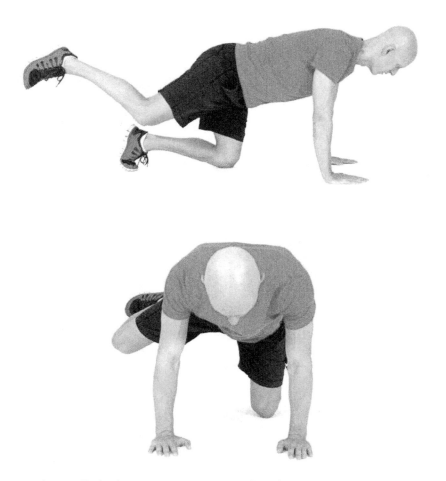

Breathing: Inhale as you prepare for the movement, and exhale as you lift your knee out to the side. Maintain a steady breathing pattern throughout the workout.

Repetitions and sets: Start with a comfortable number of repetitions, such as 8 to 10 on each side. Gradually increase the repetitions as you become more comfortable and stronger. Aim for 2 to 3 sets of the workout.

Modifications: If you find it challenging to maintain your balance or perform the workout on all fours, you can modify it by performing the workout while standing. Stand tall with your feet hip-width apart and lift one leg out to the side, like the movement of a fire hydrant. You can also increase the difficulty by adding ankle weights or resistance bands around your thighs.

Standing Hip Circles

Starting position: Stand tall with your feet hip-width apart, maintaining good posture. Place your hands on your hips or hold onto a sturdy object for balance if needed.

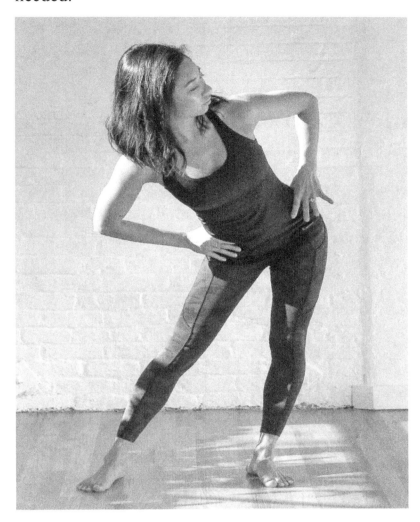

Movement description: Keep both of your feet on the ground and toes pointing forward. Begin to make circular motions with your hip. Imagine drawing a circle with your hip as the center point. Keep the movement controlled and smooth.

Breathing: Breathe naturally throughout the workout. Inhale as you start the circle, and exhale as you complete each rotation.

Repetitions and sets: Start with a comfortable number of repetitions, such as 8-10 circles in each direction. Gradually increase the number of repetitions as you become more comfortable and stronger. Aim for 2-3 sets of the workout.

Modifications: If you find it challenging to maintain balance, you can hold onto a sturdy object for support. As you gain strength and stability, you can gradually increase the size of the circles or perform the workout without holding onto any support.

Ankle and Foot Strengthening

Strong and stable ankles and feet are essential for maintaining balance, mobility, and overall functional fitness, especially for seniors. In the following workouts, we will target the muscles, tendons, and ligaments of the ankles and feet. These workouts can help improve ankle mobility, increase foot arch strength, and enhance proprioception (awareness of body positioning).

Toe Raises

Starting Position: Stand tall with your feet hip-width apart, maintaining a stable posture.

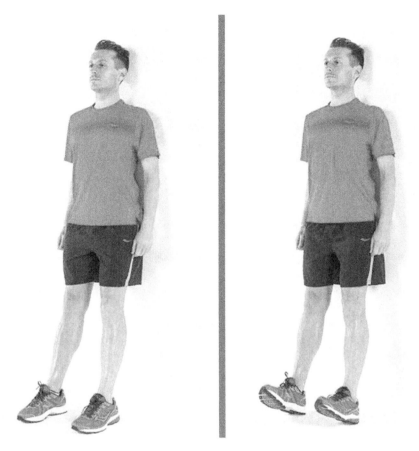

Movement Description: Slowly lift your toes off the ground while keeping your heels planted firmly. Lift your toes as high as you comfortably can, feeling the stretch in your calves and the balls of your feet. Hold the raised position for a moment, then lower your toes back down to the ground.

Breathing: Inhale as you raise your toes, and exhale as you lower them.

Repetitions and Sets: Start with 10 repetitions and gradually increase the number as you become more comfortable and stronger. Aim for 2-3 sets of toe raises.

Modifications: If you find it challenging to balance or perform the workout while standing, you can hold onto a sturdy surface for support, such as a chair or wall. As you progress, you can increase the difficulty by performing the workout on one leg at a time.

Ankle Alphabet

Starting Position: Sit on a chair with your back straight and feet flat on the ground.

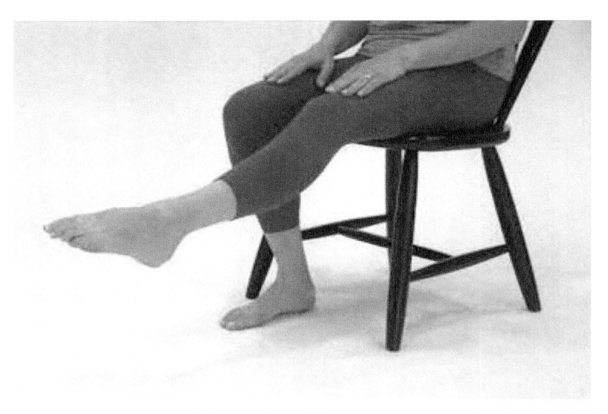

Movement Description: Lift one foot off the ground and imagine drawing the letters of the alphabet with your toes in the air. Start with the letter A and move through the entire alphabet.

Breathing: Maintain relaxed breathing throughout the workout.

Repetitions and Sets: Complete the alphabet sequence on each foot, moving smoothly and deliberately through each letter.

Modifications: If sitting on a chair is challenging, you can lie down on your back and perform the ankle alphabet with your leg elevated. You can also use your finger to trace the letters on your ankle if it's difficult to visualize.

Big Toe Stretch

Starting Position: Sit on a chair with your feet flat on the ground.

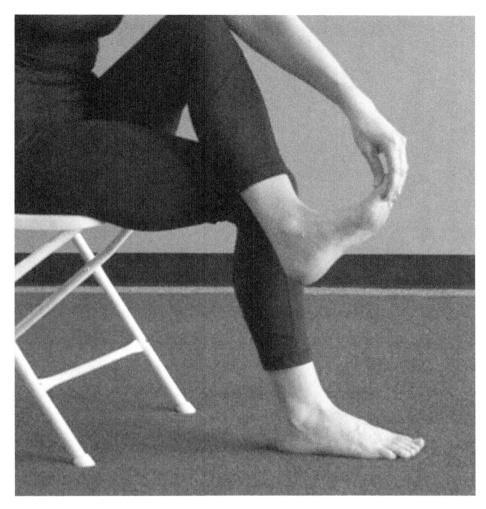

Movement Description: Lift your right foot off the ground and cross it over your left thigh, so your right ankle rests on your left knee. Interlace your fingers and place them behind your left thigh, gently pulling it towards your chest.

Duration: Hold the stretch for 20-30 seconds on each foot.

Repetitions and Sets: Perform 2-3 sets on each foot.

Modifications: If reaching your foot is difficult, you can use a towel or strap to loop around the arch of your foot and gently pull it towards you. As you progress, you can increase the duration of the stretch and the number of sets.

Marble Pick-Up

Starting Position: Sit on a chair with a small bowl of marbles on the ground in front of you.

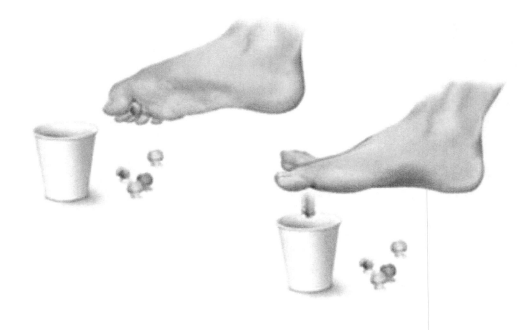

Movement Description: Use your toes to pick up the marbles, one at a time, and place them into another bowl. Focus on gripping the marbles with your toes and using the muscles in your feet and ankles to lift them.

Breathing: Maintain relaxed breathing throughout the workout. Breathe in a natural and controlled manner.

Repetitions and Sets: Start with 5-10 marbles and gradually increase the number as you improve. Aim to complete a set of picking up all the marbles from one bowl and transferring them to the other.

Modifications and Progressions: If you find it challenging to sit on a chair, you can perform this workout while lying down on your back. Place the marbles on the floor next to you and use your toes to pick them up and place them into a container by your side. This modification allows you to focus solely on the foot and ankle movements without the need for sitting.

Heel Walk

Starting Position: Stand tall with your feet together.

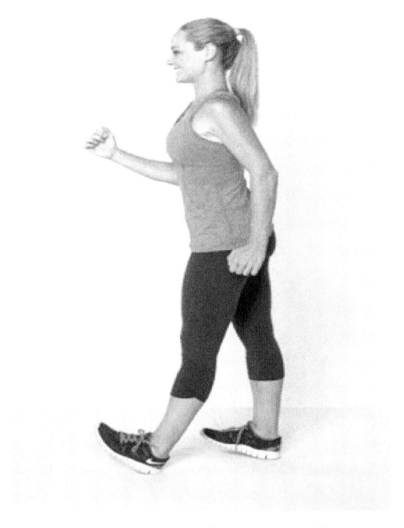

Movement Description: Lift your toes off the ground and walk forward using only your heels. Keep your toes pointed upward throughout the movement.

Repetitions and Sets: Begin by walking for 10-20 steps. As you progress, gradually increase the number of steps or distance covered.

Modifications: If you find it challenging to maintain balance or stability while walking on your heels, you can hold onto a stable surface, such as a wall or countertop, for support. As you gain strength and confidence, try performing the workout without any support.

5. CORE STABILITY AND BALANCE

Your core is more than just your abdominal muscles. It encompasses a complex network of muscles, including the abdominals, back muscles, hip muscles, and pelvic floor muscles. Building a strong and stable core is essential for maintaining proper posture, supporting your spine, and improving overall functional movement.

In this chapter, we will delve into the fundamental aspects of core strength and balance training, two key elements for maintaining a strong and stable body as we age. We will explore a range of workouts and techniques specifically designed to target and strengthen your core muscles.

Core Strengthening Workouts

Your core muscles play a crucial role in supporting your spine, maintaining proper posture, and facilitating efficient movement throughout your daily activities. Let's journey through a range of core strengthening workouts that target the deep muscles of your abdomen, back, and hips.

Building a strong core is not only about achieving a toned midsection but also about developing the functional strength necessary for everyday movements and activities. As you progress through these workouts, you will notice improvements in your posture, stability, and overall body control.

Dead Bug

Starting position:

Lie on your back on a comfortable mat or floor.

Bend your knees and lift them up, so your knees are positioned directly over your hips. Your lower legs should be parallel to the floor.

Raise your arms straight up toward the ceiling, with your wrists directly above your shoulders. This is your starting position.

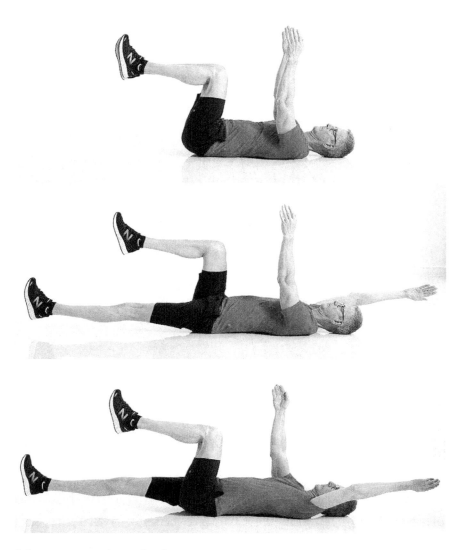

Movement description:

Engage your core muscles by gently drawing your belly button toward your spine.

Slowly and simultaneously lower your right arm behind your head and straighten your left leg, lowering it toward the floor. Keep your lower back pressed into the mat.

Pause for a moment when your arm and leg are fully extended but not touching the ground.

Slowly return your right arm and left leg back to the starting position.

Repeat the movement on the opposite side, lowering your left arm and right leg while keeping the core engaged.

Continue alternating sides for the desired number of repetitions.

Breathing:

Breathe naturally throughout the workout. Inhale as you prepare for the movement, and exhale as you extend your arm and leg away from your body. Inhale again as you return to the starting position.

Repetitions and sets:

Start with a manageable number of repetitions, such as 8-10 on each side. Gradually increase the repetitions as you become more comfortable and stronger. Aim for 2-3 sets of the workout.

Modifications:

If lifting both arms and legs simultaneously is challenging, you can begin by practicing the workout with just one arm and one leg extended at a time.

To make the workout more challenging, you can try fully extending your arm and leg closer to the ground without touching it, increasing the range of motion. .

Standing Side Bend

Starting position: Stand tall with your feet hip-width apart. Keep your arms relaxed by your sides or place your hands on your hips for added support.

Movement description: Begin by gently tilting your upper body to the right side, maintaining a straight line from your head to your hips. Keep your shoulders aligned with your hips and avoid leaning forward or backward. You should feel a stretch along the left side of your torso. Return to the starting position and then repeat the movement, this time tilting your upper body to the left side.

Breathing: Inhale as you prepare for the movement, and exhale as you tilt your upper body to the side. Continue to breathe naturally throughout the workout.

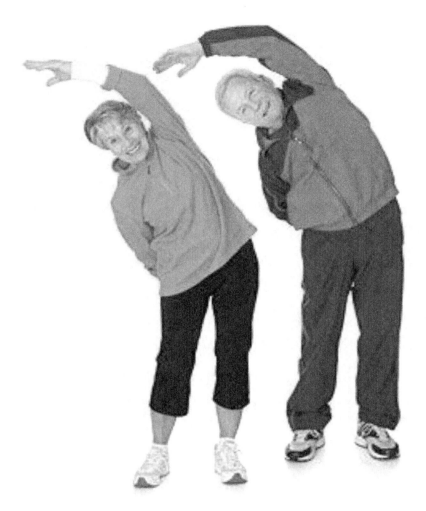

Repetitions and sets: Start with a comfortable number of repetitions, such as 8 to 10 repetitions per side. Aim to gradually increase the number of repetitions or sets as your strength and comfort level improve.

Modifications: If you find it challenging to maintain balance or experience discomfort, you can modify the workout by performing it while seated on a stable chair.

Russian Twist

Starting position: Sit on the ground with your knees bent and feet lifted off the floor. Lean back slightly, engaging your core muscles.

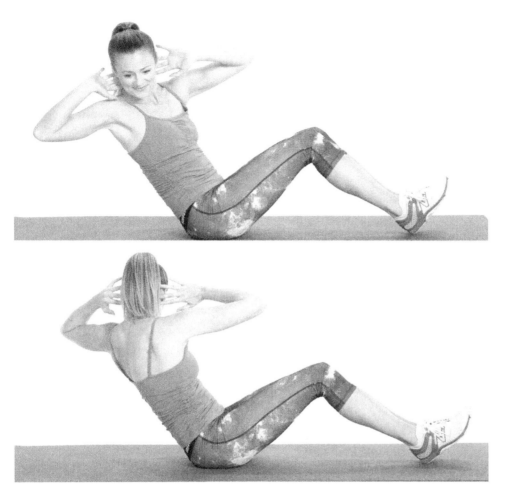

Movement description:

Extend your arms straight in front of you, interlacing your fingers or clasping your hands together.

Keeping your spine straight and your core engaged, twist your torso to the right side.

As you twist, aim to touch the ground with your hands or fingertips beside your hip. Keep your arms parallel to the ground throughout the movement.

Slowly return to the starting position and then twist your torso to the left side, aiming to touch the ground with your hands or fingertips beside your hip.

Breathing:

Remember to breathe throughout the workout. Inhale deeply before you start the twist, and exhale as you rotate your torso. Maintain a controlled and steady breathing pattern.

Start with a manageable number of repetitions, such as 8 to 10 twists on each side. Gradually increase the number of repetitions as you become more comfortable and stronger. Aim for 2 to 3 sets of Russian Twists during your workout session.

Modifications:

To make the workout easier: Keep your feet on the ground instead of lifting them off. You can also choose to perform smaller twists with less range of motion.

Supine Leg Lifts

Starting Position:

Lie on your back on a mat or comfortable surface.

Extend your legs fully and place your arms alongside your body, palms facing down.

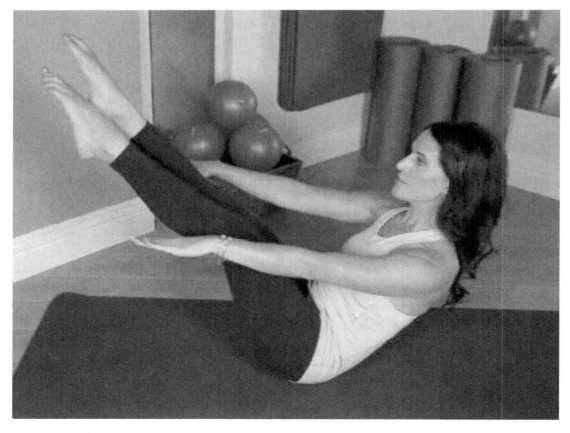

Movement Description:

Keeping your legs straight, slowly lift both legs off the ground simultaneously.

Continue lifting until your legs are at a 45-degree angle or as high as you comfortably can go.

Hold the lifted position briefly, engaging your core muscles.

Breathing:

Breathe in as you lower your legs towards the ground.

Breathe out as you lift your legs back up.

Repetitions and Sets:

Start with a comfortable number of repetitions, such as 8-10.

Gradually increase the number of repetitions as you get stronger.

Aim for 2-3 sets of this workout.

Modifications:

To make this workout easier, you can bend your knees slightly or lift one leg at a time instead of both legs simultaneously.

Standing March

Starting position:

Stand tall with your feet hip-width apart.

Keep your shoulders relaxed and maintain good posture throughout the workout.

Engage your core by drawing your belly button in towards your spine.

Movement description:

Lift one knee up towards your chest while keeping your core engaged.

Slowly lower the lifted leg back down to the starting position.

Repeat the same movement with the opposite leg.

Continue alternating between the right and left legs in a marching motion.

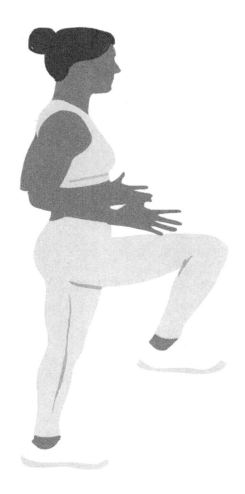

Repetitions and sets:

Start with a comfortable number of repetitions and sets based on your fitness level. Beginners can begin with 10 to 12 repetitions on each leg and gradually increase as they become more comfortable and stronger. Aim for 1 to 3 sets of the workout.

Modifications:

If standing for the entire duration is challenging, you can perform the workout while seated on a stable chair.

To increase the challenge, you can add arm movements by swinging your opposite arm forward as you lift your knee.

Flutter Kicks

Starting position:

Lie on your back on a comfortable surface such as a mat or carpet.

Extend your legs fully, keeping them close together.

Place your arms by your sides, palms facing down, for support.

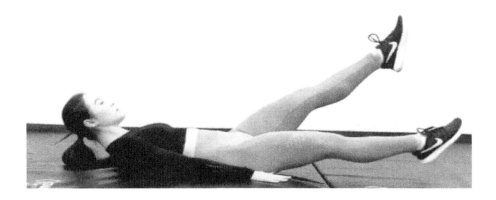

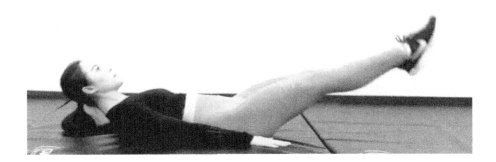

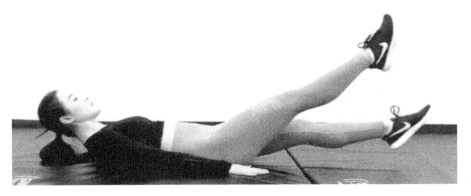

Movement description:

Lift both legs a few inches off the ground, maintaining a slight bend in your knees.

Keep your core engaged and your lower back pressed against the floor or mat throughout the workout.

Begin alternating small, quick movements of your legs up and down in a scissor-like motion.

Make sure to keep your legs straight and toes pointed during the movement.

Breathing:

Breathe naturally throughout the workout, inhaling and exhaling at a comfortable pace.

Avoid holding your breath and maintain a relaxed breathing pattern.

Repetitions and sets:

Start with a manageable number of repetitions, such as 10 to 15 flutter kicks.

Aim to gradually increase the number of repetitions over time as your strength and endurance improve.

Perform 2 to 3 sets of flutter kicks, resting briefly between sets.

Modifications:

If you find it challenging to keep your legs fully extended, you can slightly bend your knees to reduce the difficulty.

Alternatively, if you want to increase the intensity, you can extend your legs closer to the ground without touching it.

Bicycle Crunches

Starting position:

Lie on your back on a comfortable mat or floor.

Bend your knees and lift your feet off the ground, so your legs form a 90-degree angle.

Place your hands lightly behind your head, elbows out to the sides.

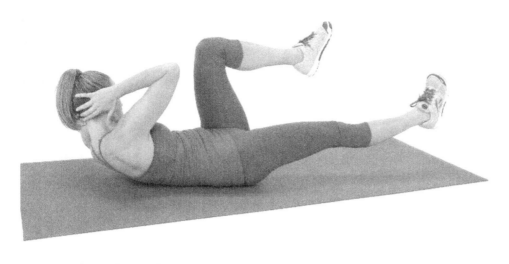

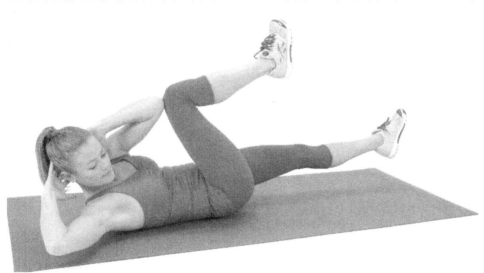

Movement description:

Engage your core muscles by drawing your belly button in towards your spine.

Lift your shoulder blades off the ground, bringing your upper body towards your knees.

Simultaneously, straighten your right leg and bring your left knee in towards your chest.

Twist your upper body to the left, aiming to bring your right elbow towards your left knee.

Hold this position for a moment, feeling the contraction in your abdominal muscles.

Slowly reverse the movement by straightening your left leg and bringing your right knee in towards your chest.

Twist your upper body to the right, aiming to bring your left elbow towards your right knee.

Hold this position briefly before repeating the movement.

Repetitions and sets:

Start with a comfortable number of repetitions, such as 10 to 15 on each side, and gradually increase as you build strength and endurance. Aim for 2 to 3 sets of bicycle crunches.

Modifications:

For beginners or those with limited mobility, you can perform the workout with smaller movements, focusing on the twisting motion while keeping the legs closer to the ground.

To increase the intensity, you can perform the workout at a slower tempo, pause for longer at the top position, or incorporate a resistance band around your thighs for added resistance.

Modified Plank

Starting position:

Begin on your knees and forearms, with your elbows aligned under your shoulders.

Place your forearms parallel to each other on the ground, shoulder-width apart.

Keep your knees together and rest on the ground, forming a 90-degree angle with your legs.

Movement description:

Straighten your legs and lift your knees off the ground, balancing on your toes and forearms.

Maintain a straight line from your head to your heels, engaging your core muscles.

Keep your back flat and avoid raising your hips too high or letting them sag.

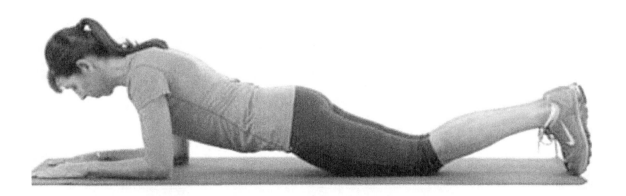

Breathing:

Focus on maintaining a steady and controlled breathing pattern throughout the workout. Inhale deeply through your nose and exhale slowly through your mouth.

Repetitions and sets:

Start with holding the position for 10 to 20 seconds, gradually increasing the duration as you build strength and stability. Aim for 2 to 3 sets of repetitions.

Modifications:

If the full Modified Plank is too challenging initially, you can keep your knees on the ground and perform the workout with the same form and alignment.

As you progress, you can increase the duration of each hold, aiming for 30 seconds or more.

For an added challenge, you can lift one leg or arm off the ground while maintaining a stable plank position.

Mountain Climbers

Starting Position:

Begin in a high plank position with your hands directly under your shoulders and your body forming a straight line from head to heels.

Engage your core muscles by drawing your belly button towards your spine.

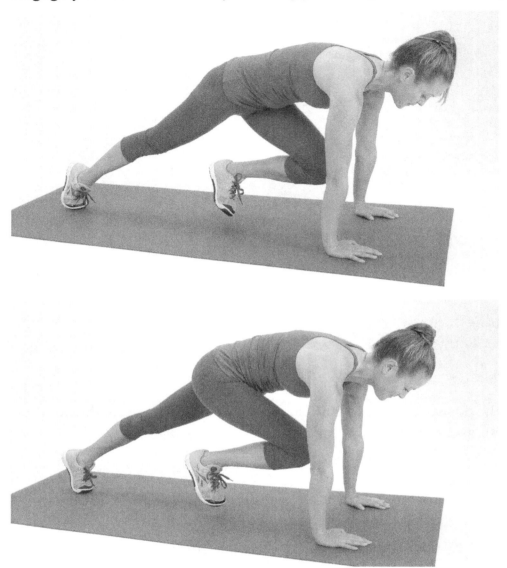

Movement Description:

Begin by bringing one knee towards your chest, keeping your foot off the ground.

Quickly switch legs, extending the first leg back while simultaneously bringing the other knee towards your chest.

Continue alternating legs in a running motion, as if you are climbing a mountain.

Maintain a controlled and steady pace throughout the workout.

Repetitions and Sets:

Start with a comfortable number of repetitions, such as 10 to 15, and gradually increase as your strength and endurance improve.

Aim to complete 2 to 3 sets of mountain climbers with short rest periods in between.

Modifications:

If the high plank position is challenging, you can modify the workout by performing mountain climbers from a kneeling plank position, with your knees resting on the ground.

As you become more comfortable, increase the speed of your leg movements, elevating the intensity of the workout.

Alternatively, you can perform mountain climbers on an elevated surface, such as a bench or step, to decrease the amount of weight bearing on your upper body.

Balance Training

Balance training is an essential component of any well-rounded fitness routine, and it becomes even more crucial as we age. Maintaining good balance not only helps prevent falls and injuries but also enhances overall stability and confidence in daily activities. Let's explore some balance workouts for you.

Flamingo Stand

Starting position: Begin by standing tall with your feet hip-width apart.

Movement description: Lift one leg off the ground and bend it at the knee, bringing your foot up towards your buttocks. Hold this position, balancing on the standing leg.

Repetitions and sets: Aim to hold the Flamingo Stand for about 30 seconds on each leg. Start with one set on each leg and gradually increase the duration as your balance improves.

Modifications: If you're new to balance workouts or have difficulty maintaining stability, you can perform the Flamingo Stand while lightly holding onto a sturdy chair or wall for support. As you become more confident and stable, gradually reduce your reliance on the support and work towards performing the workout without assistance.

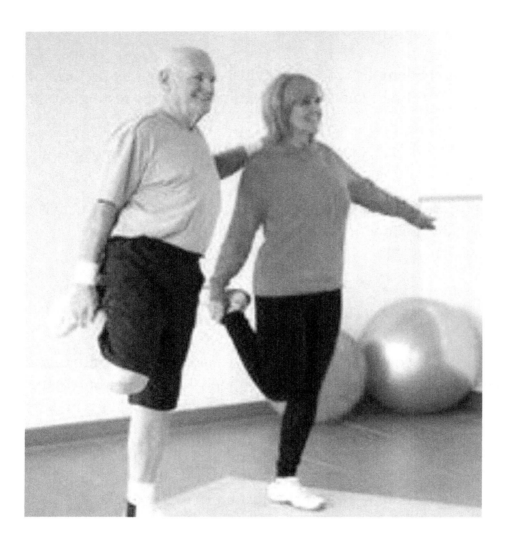

Clock Reach

Starting Position:

Stand on one leg with your feet hip-width apart and your core engaged.

Find a focal point in front of you to help with balance.

Movement Description:

Imagine there is a clock on the floor in front of you.

Lift your free leg slightly off the ground and maintain your balance on the standing leg.

Begin reaching your free leg to different clock positions.

For example, start by reaching your leg forward to 12 o'clock, then return it to the starting position.

Next, reach your leg out to the side to 3 o'clock, and return to the starting position.

Finally, reach your leg backward to 6 o'clock, and return to the starting position.

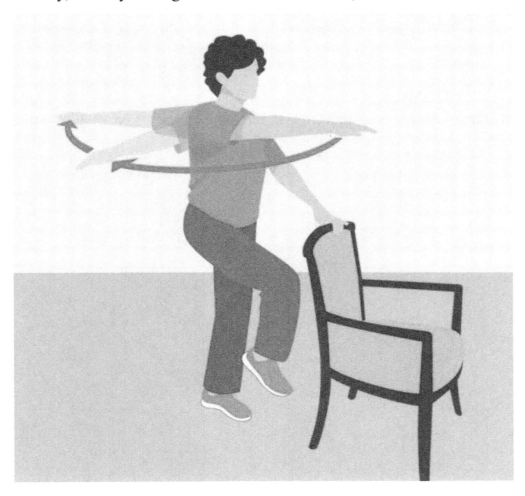

Repetitions and Sets:

Aim to perform 5-10 repetitions of the clock reach workout on each leg.

Start with a lower number of repetitions and gradually increase as your balance and confidence improve.

You can perform multiple sets of this workout, depending on your fitness level and comfort.

Modifications:

If you're just starting or have limited balance, you can lightly touch a wall or sturdy support for assistance.

As you gain stability, try performing the workout without support.

To increase the challenge, you can extend the reach of your leg further or hold each clock position for a few seconds before returning to the starting position.

Yoga Tree Pose

Starting Position: Stand tall with your feet hip-width apart and arms relaxed by your sides.

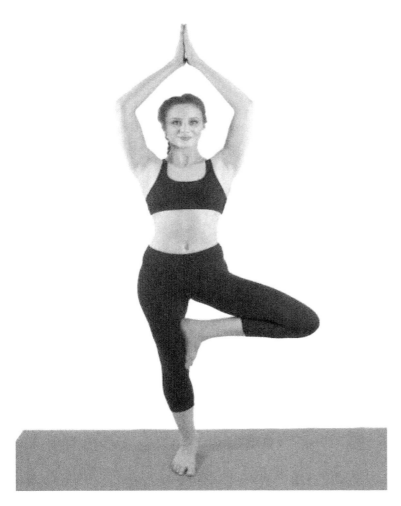

Movement Description:

Shift your weight onto your left foot and lift your right foot off the ground.

Place the sole of your right foot on the inner thigh of your left leg, either above or below the knee. Avoid placing it directly on the knee joint.

Find your balance and engage your core muscles to help stabilize your body.

Bring your hands together in front of your chest in a prayer position or extend your arms overhead for an added challenge.

Find a focal point in front of you to help maintain your balance and focus.

Breathing:

Breathe deeply and evenly throughout the workout, inhaling and exhaling slowly. Focus on maintaining relaxed and steady breath to help center your mind and improve your balance.

Repetitions and Sets:

Hold the Yoga Tree Pose for about 30 seconds to 1 minute on each leg. Start with a shorter duration if needed and gradually increase the time as your balance improves. Repeat the workout 2 to 3 times on each leg.

Modifications:

If you have difficulty balancing, you can place the sole of your foot on the inner calf or ankle of your standing leg instead of the thigh.

For additional support, you can lightly touch a wall or sturdy object with your fingertips.

To challenge yourself further, try closing your eyes while maintaining the pose. This increases the reliance on your proprioception, or the body's sense of its position in space, to enhance balance.

Tandem Stance

Starting Position:

Stand tall with your feet together, arms relaxed by your sides.

Choose a fixed point in front of you to focus your gaze on, which will help with your balance.

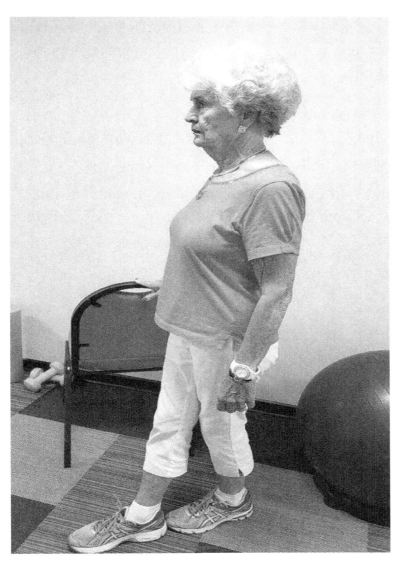

Movement Description:

Lift one foot and place it directly in front of the other foot, so that your heel is touching the toes of your opposite foot.

Keep your arms relaxed by your sides or gently place your hands on your hips for added stability.

Engage your core muscles to maintain an upright posture and a steady stance.

Try to distribute your weight evenly between both feet, finding your center of balance.

Repetitions and Sets:

Hold the tandem stance for 30 seconds to start with, or if you can comfortably maintain your balance. Gradually increase the duration as your balance improves. Aim to perform 2 to 3 sets of workouts.

Modifications:

If you're finding it challenging to balance, you can lightly touch a wall, countertop, or sturdy chair for support until you feel more confident.

To progress the workout, try closing your eyes while maintaining the tandem stance. This will further challenge your balance and proprioception (awareness of your body's position in space).

Standing Knee Lifts

Starting Position:

Stand tall with your feet hip-width apart and arms relaxed by Description

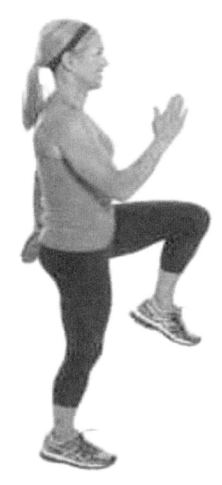

Movement Description:

Engage your core and maintain good posture throughout the workout.

Lift one knee towards your chest while keeping your foot flexed.

Slowly lower the lifted leg back down to the starting position.

Repeat the movement with the opposite leg.

Continue alternating legs, lifting one knee at a time.

Breathing:

Inhale as you lift your knee towards your chest and exhale as you lower your leg back down.

Repetitions and Sets:

Start with a comfortable number of repetitions, such as 5-10 on each leg. Gradually increase the number of repetitions as you become more comfortable and confident with the workout. Aim for 2-3 sets.

Modifications:

If you have difficulty lifting your knee all the way to your chest, start by lifting it as high as you can comfortably manage and gradually work towards a higher range of motion.

If you need additional support, you can hold onto a sturdy surface, such as a chair or wall, while performing the workout.

To increase the challenge, you can incorporate variations such as holding the knee lift for a few seconds or adding a small hop while switching legs.

One-Legged Balance Reach

Starting Position:

Stand on one leg, keeping your body upright and your core engaged.

Find a focal point in front of you to help maintain your balance.

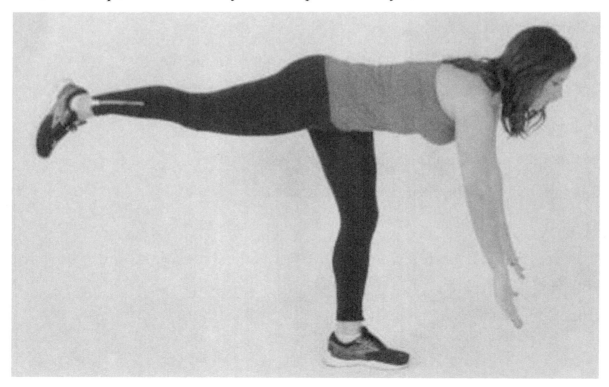

Movement Description:

Slowly lean forward from your hips, while extending your opposite leg straight behind you.

Keep your standing knee slightly bent and your back straight.

Reach forward with your arms, maintaining a strong and controlled movement.

Aim to bring your extended leg and torso parallel to the ground, forming a straight line.

Keep your gaze focused ahead to assist with balance and stability.

Breathing:

Breathe steadily throughout the workout. Inhale deeply before initiating the movement, and exhale as you lean forward and extend your leg behind you. Maintain a controlled and rhythmic breathing pattern.

Repetitions and Sets:

Start with 5-10 repetitions on each leg, gradually increasing the number as you gain strength and stability. Aim for 2-3 sets of the workout.

Modifications:

If you find it challenging to maintain balance, you can lightly touch a wall or stable surface with your fingertips for support.

To make the workout easier, you can reduce the range of motion and only lean forward slightly while keeping your back leg closer to the ground.

To progress the workout, increase the duration of the hold at the bottom position, or try closing your eyes to further challenge your balance.

Single-Leg Stance

Starting position: Stand tall with your feet hip-width apart, arms relaxed by your sides, and your gaze forward.

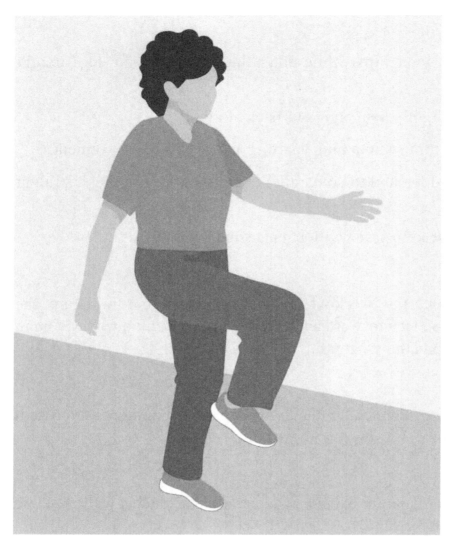

Movement description: Lift one foot off the ground, bending your knee slightly, and balance on the other leg. Keep your posture upright and engage your core for stability.

Repetitions and sets: Start by holding the single-leg stance for 20-30 seconds on each leg. As you become more comfortable and confident, gradually increase the duration to challenge your balance. Aim for 2-3 sets on each leg.

Modifications: If you find it difficult to balance on one leg, you can use a sturdy chair or wall for support. Lightly place your fingertips on the support while still engaging your leg muscles to maintain balance. As you build strength and stability, aim to reduce the reliance on the support and eventually perform the workout without assistance.

Cross-Body Toe Touches

Starting position: Stand tall with your feet hip-width apart, maintaining good posture and balance.

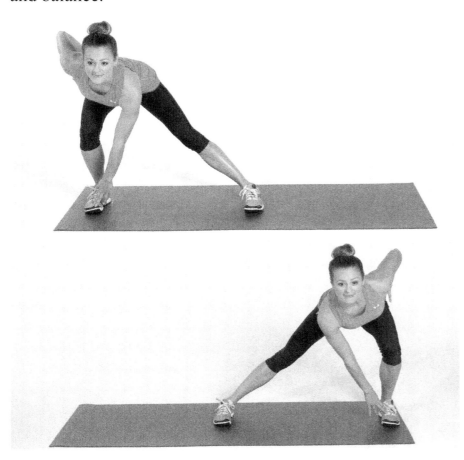

Movement description: Lift one leg off the ground, bending your knee slightly for stability. Simultaneously, reach down with the opposite hand and try to touch your toes on the lifted leg. Keep your core engaged and maintain a steady balance throughout the movement. Return to the starting position and repeat on the other side.

Repetitions and sets: Start with a comfortable number of repetitions, such as 8-10 on each side. Gradually increase the repetitions or sets as you feel more confident and balanced.

Modifications: If you're just starting out or have balance concerns, you can perform the workout near a wall or sturdy chair to provide support. Instead of lifting your leg high, you can begin with smaller movements, like knee raises or reaching toward your shin. As you progress, aim to increase the range of motion and challenge your balance by lifting your leg higher and reaching closer to your toes.

6. FLEXIBILITY AND RANGE OF MOTION

Flexibility is not just about touching your toes or performing impressive contortions; it's about achieving functional mobility that allows you to perform daily tasks with ease and grace. Whether it's bending down to tie your shoes, reaching for objects on high shelves, or simply enjoying a pain-free range of motion, flexibility training can significantly enhance your quality of life.

In this chapter, we will explore various stretching techniques, including static stretches, dynamic stretches, and mobility workouts, ensuring that you not only improve your flexibility but also maintain joint health and prevent muscle imbalances.

Full-Body Stretches

The stretches we will cover encompass various areas of the body, including the neck, shoulders, back, hips, and legs. Each stretch is carefully selected to target specific muscle groups and improve flexibility in those areas.

Neck Stretch

Starting Position: Sit tall with your spine straight, either on a chair or on the floor.

Movement Description: Slowly tilt your head to one side, bringing your ear toward your shoulder. Keep your shoulders relaxed and avoid shrugging them up. You should feel a gentle stretch on the side of your neck. Hold this position for a few seconds.

Breathing: Take deep, slow breaths while performing the stretch. Inhale as you prepare, and exhale as you tilt your head to the side.

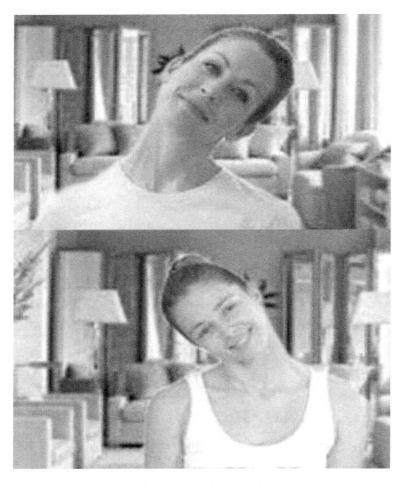

Repetitions and Sets: Perform the stretch on one side, holding for around 10-15 seconds. Repeat the stretch on the other side, ensuring you maintain the same duration. Aim for 2-3 sets on each side.

Modifications: If you have limited range of motion, you can modify the stretch by reducing the range of the head tilt.

Shoulder Stretch

Starting Position: Stand or sit in a comfortable position with your spine straight and your feet shoulder-width apart.

Movement Description: Extend one arm straight out in front of you at shoulder height. Keep your palm facing down. Slowly bring your extended arm across your body towards the opposite shoulder, allowing your shoulder to rotate inward. Feel a gentle stretch in your shoulder and upper back. Hold the stretch for a few seconds.

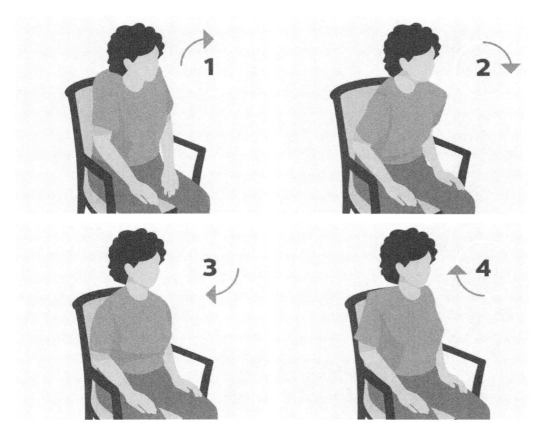

Repetitions and Sets: Perform this stretch 2-3 times on each side, holding each stretch for about 10-15 seconds. Repeat as desired or needed.

Modifications:

If you have limited mobility in your shoulders, you can start by performing the stretch with a smaller range of motion. Gradually increase the range of motion as your flexibility improves.

To deepen the stretch, you can use your other hand to gently pull your extended arm closer to your body.

If standing is challenging, you can perform this stretch while seated. Simply sit tall with your feet flat on the ground and follow the same movement description

Spinal Twist

Starting Position: Sit on a chair with your feet flat on the ground, maintaining an upright posture. Place your hands on your thighs or hold onto the sides of the chair for support.

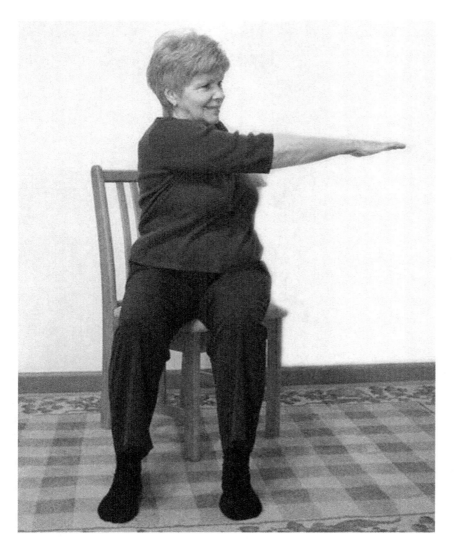

Movement Description: Take a deep breath in and as you exhale, gently twist your upper body to one side. Place one hand on the outside of the opposite knee and the other hand on the back of the chair. Use the support of your hands to assist the twist.

Breathing: Breathe deeply and comfortably throughout the stretch. Inhale to prepare, and as you exhale, allow your body to twist a little further, deepening the stretch.

Repetitions and Sets: Hold the twist for about 15 to 30 seconds, feeling a gentle stretch in your back. Release the twist and return to the starting position. Repeat the stretch on the other side.

Modifications: If you have limited mobility or flexibility, you can modify the stretch by twisting your upper body to a comfortable range.

Hip Flexor Stretch

Starting Position: Stand near a wall or hold onto a sturdy surface for support.

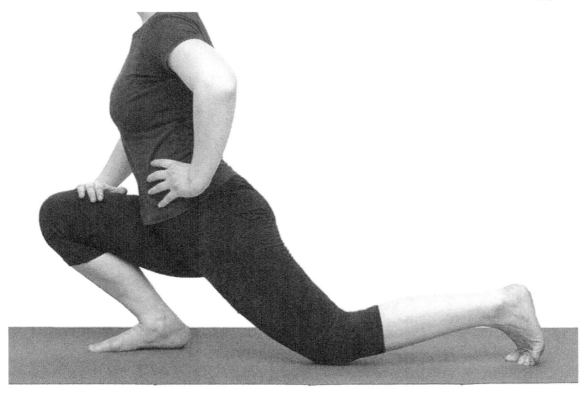

Movement Description: Take a step back with one leg, creating a lunge position. Ensure that your front knee is directly above your ankle and your back leg is extended. Keep your upper body upright and engage your core muscles for stability.

Repetitions and Sets: Hold the stretch for 20 to 30 seconds on each side. Repeat the stretch 2 to 3 times on each leg.

Modifications: If you have difficulty maintaining balance, you can perform this stretch while holding onto a sturdy chair or wall for support. To increase the intensity of the stretch, you can slightly tilt your pelvis forward, emphasizing the stretch in the hip flexor.

Hamstring Stretch

Starting Position: Sit on the edge of a chair with your feet flat on the floor, hip-width apart. Sit up tall with a straight spine and relax your shoulders.

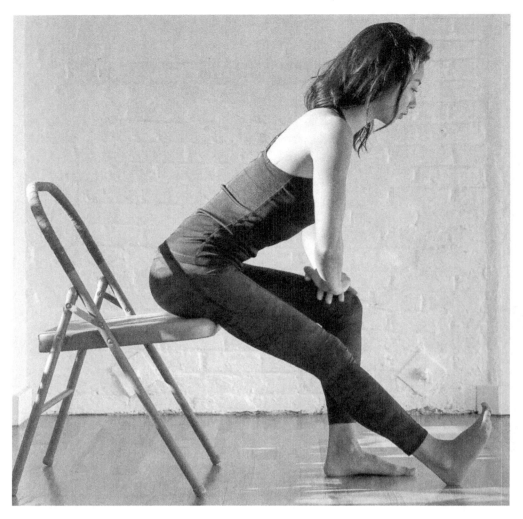

Movement Description: Extend one leg out in front of you, resting your heel on the floor. Keep your toes pointing upward. Slowly lean forward from your hips, reaching toward your toes. Maintain a slight bend in your knee if needed to avoid any discomfort or strain.

Repetitions and Sets: Hold the stretch for 15 to 30 seconds, feeling a gentle pull in the back of your thigh. Repeat the stretch 2 to 3 times on each leg.

Modifications: If you have difficulty reaching your toes, you can use a towel or a strap to gently pull your foot closer. Alternatively, you can perform the stretch while lying on your back, raising one leg up and supporting it with your hands behind the thigh.

Quadriceps Stretch

Starting Position: Stand near a wall or hold onto a sturdy surface for support.

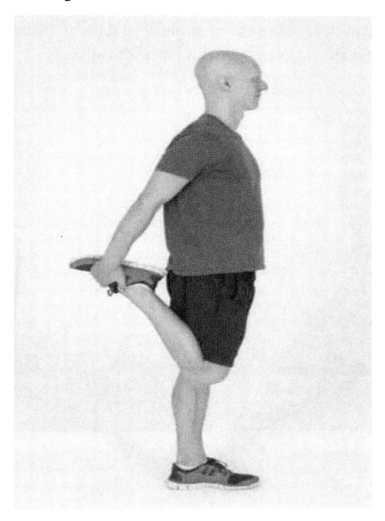

Movement Description: Bend one knee and grasp your ankle, bringing your heel towards your buttocks. Keep your knees close together and maintain an upright posture.

Repetitions and Sets: Hold the stretch for about 15 to 30 seconds on each leg. Repeat the stretch 2 to 3 times on each side.

Modifications: If it's challenging to reach your ankle, you can use a towel or strap to loop around your foot and hold onto that for support. As you become more flexible, you can gradually increase the intensity of the stretch by gently pulling your heel closer to your buttocks.

Calf Stretch

Starting Position: Stand facing a wall or hold onto a sturdy surface for support. Place your hands on the wall at shoulder height and keep your feet hip-width apart.

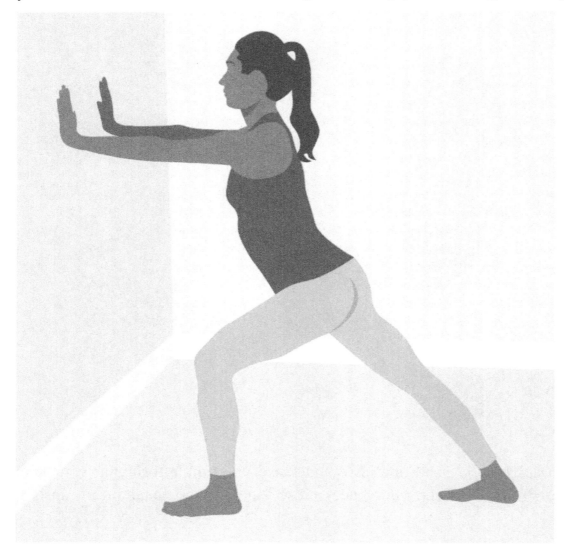

Movement Description: Step one foot back, keeping it straight with the heel on the ground. Keep your front knee slightly bent. Lean forward by shifting your weight onto your front foot, while keeping your back leg straight. You should feel a stretch in your calf muscle.

Repetitions and Sets: Hold the stretch for about 20-30 seconds, feeling a gentle pulling sensation in your calf muscle. Repeat the stretch 2-3 times on each leg.

Modifications: If you find it challenging to maintain balance while standing, you can perform this stretch while sitting on a chair. Extend one leg out in front of you with the heel on the ground and lean forward from your hips, feeling the stretch in your calf. You can also progress the stretch by placing a slight bend in your front knee, which will increase the intensity of the stretch.

Inner Thigh Stretch

Starting position: Sit on the edge of a chair with your back straight and feet together.

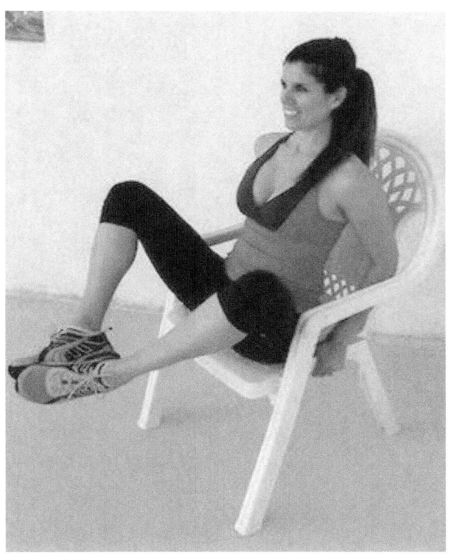

Movement description: Allow your knees to fall outward, creating a diamond shape with your legs. Keep your feet touching each other and your heels close to your body.

Repetitions and sets: Hold the stretch for 15 to 30 seconds, feeling a gentle pull in your inner thighs. Repeat the stretch for a total of 2 to 3 times.

Modifications: If you have difficulty maintaining the position, you can place a folded towel or cushion under each knee for support. As you become more comfortable with the stretch, you can increase the duration of each repetition or try extending your legs a little wider for a deeper stretch.

Glute Stretch

Starting Position:

Begin by lying on your back with your knees bent and feet flat on the floor.

Cross your left ankle over your right knee.

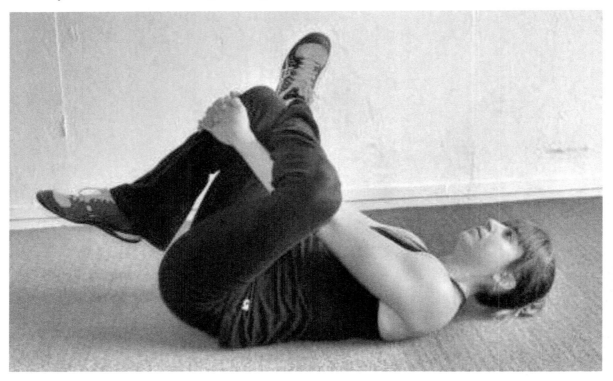

Movement Description:

Gently pull your right knee towards your chest, while keeping your left foot flexed.

Hold the stretch for 15-30 seconds, feeling a stretch in your left glute and hip.

Repeat on the other side, crossing your right ankle over your left knee and pulling your left knee towards your chest.

Repetitions and Sets:

Hold each stretch for 15-30 seconds on each side and repeat the stretch 2-3 times on each side.

Modifications:

If you find it difficult to reach your knee, you can use a towel or a yoga strap to help pull your leg closer to your chest. To increase the intensity of the stretch, you can lift your head and shoulders off the ground and bring your nose towards your knee, deepening the stretch in your glutes.

Bonus Workout

Side-to-Side Steps

Starting Position:

Stand with your feet hip-width apart, keeping your posture tall and your core engaged. Place your hands on your hips or allow them to hang naturally by your sides.

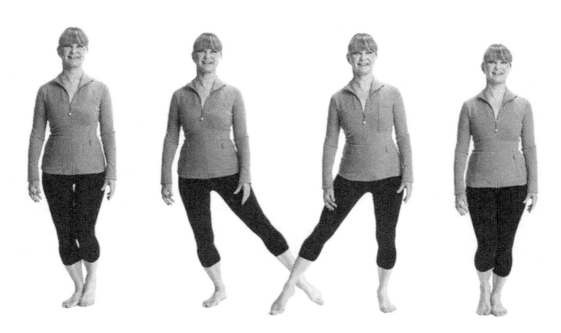

Movement Description:

Step your right foot out to the side, wider than your hips, while maintaining a slight bend in your knees. As you step, shift your body weight onto your right foot, keeping your left foot planted firmly on the ground. Then, step your left foot in to meet your right foot, returning to the starting position. Repeat the same movement pattern, this time stepping to the left side. Continue alternating side-to-side steps.

Breathing:

Inhale as you step out to the side, and exhale as you bring your feet back together. Maintain a steady and controlled breathing pattern throughout the workout.

Repetitions and Sets:

Start with a comfortable number of repetitions, such as 8 to 10 steps on each side. Gradually increase the number of repetitions as you become more comfortable and confident with the workout. Aim for 2 to 3 sets, allowing yourself a brief rest between sets.

Modifications:

If you have difficulty with balance, perform this workout while holding onto a stable surface, such as a chair or wall, for support.

For a more dynamic and challenging variation, increase the speed of your side-to-side steps, incorporating a slight hop or jump as you move from side to side.

Stair Climbing

Starting Position: Stand at the bottom of a flight of stairs with your feet hip-width apart. Place your hands on the railing or keep them relaxed by your sides, depending on your balance and stability.

Movement Description: Step onto the first step with one foot, followed by the other foot. Continue climbing the stairs by lifting one foot at a time and placing it on the next step. Maintain a steady and controlled pace throughout the workout.

Breathing: Breathe naturally throughout the workout. Inhale as you lift your foot to step onto the next stair, and exhale as you push off with your trailing foot.

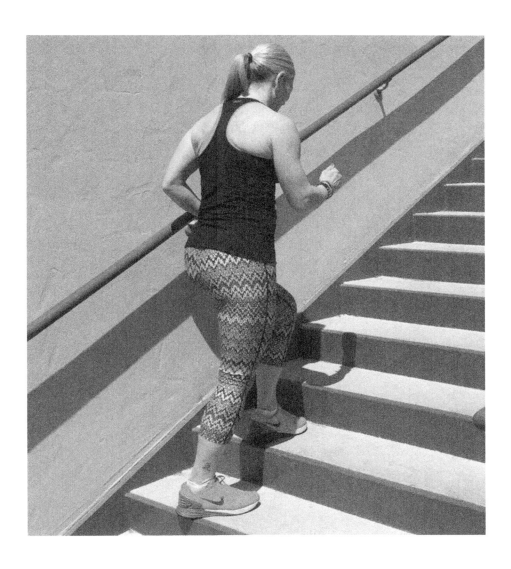

Repetitions and Sets: The number of repetitions and sets can vary depending on your fitness level and goals. Start with a comfortable number of repetitions, such as 5 to 10, and gradually increase as you build strength and endurance. Aim for 2 to 3 sets initially and progress from there.

Modifications: If you find stair climbing challenging, you can start with a shorter flight of stairs or use a single step at home. You can also hold onto a railing or use a walking aid for support and stability. To progress the workout, you can increase the number of stairs, climb at a faster pace, or add intervals of double steps or skipping steps for a more challenging workout.

Backward Stride

Starting Position: Stand tall with your feet hip-width apart, maintaining good posture. Keep your core engaged and your shoulders relaxed.

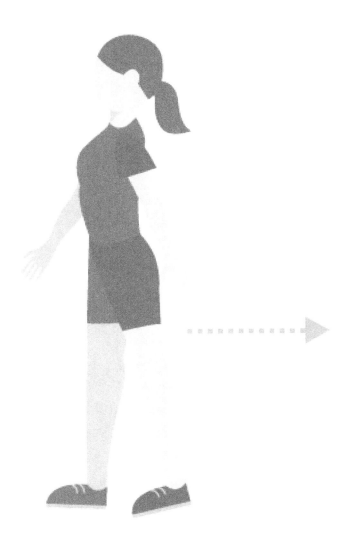

Movement Description: Step backward with one foot, extending your leg behind you. Lower your body down by bending your front knee and descending into a lunge position. Maintain a straight back and keep your chest lifted throughout the movement. The back knee can hover slightly above the ground or lightly touch the floor.

Breathing: Inhale as you step back and prepare for the movement. Exhale as you lower your body into the lunge position. Inhale again as you push through your front foot to return to the starting position.

Repetitions and Sets: Start with a comfortable number of repetitions, such as 8 to 10 per leg. Gradually increase the repetitions as your strength and stability improve. Aim for 2 to 3 sets of the workout, resting for a short period between sets.

Modifications: For beginners or those with limited mobility, the range of motion can be reduced by not descending as deeply into the lunge position. You can also use a chair or wall for support if needed. To progress the workout, you can increase the depth of the lunge, incorporate weights (such as holding dumbbells), or perform the movement at a slower pace to challenge your balance and control.

Seated Torso Twists

Starting position: Sit on a chair with your feet planted firmly on the ground. Keep your back straight and engage your core muscles for stability.

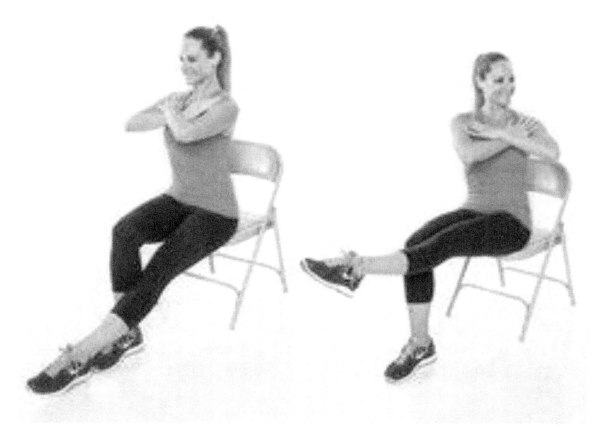

Movement description: Place your hands on your shoulders, with your elbows pointing out to the sides. Slowly twist your upper body to one side, rotating your torso from the waist. Keep your hips and lower body facing forward. Pause for a moment in the twisted position.

Breathing: Inhale before initiating the twist and exhale as you rotate your upper body to the side. Maintain a steady and controlled breathing pattern throughout the workout.

Repetitions and sets: Start with a comfortable range of motion and aim for 8-12 repetitions on each side. You can gradually increase the number of repetitions as you become more comfortable and stronger. Perform 2-3 sets of the workout, resting briefly between sets.

Modifications: If you have limited mobility or flexibility, you can reduce the range of motion and perform smaller twists. If you want to make the workout more challenging, you can hold a lightweight object, such as a small water bottle, in your hands while performing the twists.

Designing A Routine that Fits Your Lifestyle and Schedule

Designing a routine that fits your lifestyle and schedule is important, if you want the best out of your workouts and make greater use of this book. By creating a structured plan, you can ensure consistency and maximize the benefits of your workouts.

Start by assessing how much time you can dedicate to workout each day or week. Consider your other commitments and obligations to find a realistic time slot for your workouts. This will help you determine the frequency and duration of your workout sessions. Setting specific and achievable goals will guide your training and provide a sense of accomplishment.

Choose the frequency of your workouts. Aim for a minimum of three to five sessions per week to experience noticeable improvements. Spread out your workouts throughout the week for better recovery and consistency. Decide on the specific days of the week when you will engage in your bodyweight workouts. Consistency is key, so choose days that are most suitable for you and try to stick to the schedule.

Make sure to include a warm-up phase at the beginning of each session to prepare your body for the workout. Similarly, allocate time for a cool-down phase at the end of your workout to stretch and relax your muscles. Customize your routine by selecting a variety of bodyweight workouts that target different muscle groups and aspects of fitness. Include workouts for strength, flexibility, balance, and cardiovascular endurance. Mixing and matching workouts will keep your routine engaging and enjoyable.

As you progress, gradually increase the intensity of your workouts. Start with workouts that match your current fitness level and gradually progress to more challenging variations. Increase repetitions, sets, or workout difficulty as you get stronger and more comfortable with the movements. Also, listen to your body and pay attention to how it responds to the workouts. Adjust the intensity or modify the workouts if needed. Rest and recover when necessary to prevent overexertion and injury.

Conclusion: Embrace the Benefits, Embrace A Healthier You

As we reach the end of this book, we hope you feel inspired and empowered to embark on a transformative journey towards better health and well-being. Throughout these pages, we have delved into a multitude of bodyweight workouts specifically tailored for seniors, equipping you with the knowledge and tools to make positive changes in your life.

Remember, this is not just a book—it is a roadmap to help you unlock your true potential. By embracing the benefits of regular exercise and incorporating these bodyweight workouts into your daily routine, you are taking a proactive step towards a healthier and happier you.

Each workout, stretch, and movement described in this guide has been carefully designed to improve your strength, flexibility, and cardiovascular endurance. The modifications and progressions provided ensure that these workouts can be adapted to your current fitness level, allowing you to challenge yourself while respecting your body's limits.

But this journey is not just about physical transformation. It's about rediscovering the joy of movement, reclaiming your vitality, and nurturing your overall well-being. It's about taking control of your health and embracing the incredible potential that lies within you. As you embark on this extraordinary path of wellness, remember to listen to your body, be patient with yourself, and celebrate every small victory along the way. Allow this book to be your guide, providing you with the knowledge, inspiration, and support you need to succeed.

So, with commitment, determination, and a belief in your own potential, embrace the benefits that await you. Embrace a healthier you, and let the world witness the amazing transformations that unfold as you embrace this journey towards a brighter, healthier future. The power is in your hands, and we have every confidence that you will thrive. Here's to your health, vitality, and a life filled with joy and fulfillment.

Printed in Great Britain
by Amazon